AF365010

YOUR HEALTH IN YOUR HANDS

How to be healthy
in spite of "medical science"

Patrick Quanten
from interviews with Alicia Ninou

Disclaimer

Material provided in this book is designed to offer helpful, general information on a wide range of topics related to your life. This book is not meant to be used, nor should it be used, to diagnose or treat any medical condition. For diagnosis or treatment of any medical problem, consult your own physician. In addition, this book is not meant to be used for specific legal advice. For matters pertaining to law, consult a lawyer, legal aid or public interest organization.

The publisher, author and experts quoted are not responsible for any specific health or legal matters that may require professional advice or supervision and are not liable for any damages or negative consequences from any action taken by an individual reading or following the information in this book.

References are provided for informational purposes only and do not constitute endorsement of any websites or other sources. Readers should be aware that the laws, regulations and interpretations cited may change. Likewise, websites listed in this book may change. Readers should seek available resources and updates for the most current information available.

This book has not been created to be specific to any individual's or organization's situation or needs. Every effort has been made to make this book as accurate as possible. This book should serve only as a general guide and not as the ultimate source of subject information. This book contains information that might be dated and is intended only to educate and entertain. The authors shall have no liability or responsibility to any person or entity regarding any loss or damage alleged to have occurred, directly or indirectly, from the information in this book.

CONTENTS

INTRODUCTION

Patrick Quanten

I began to realise something was wrong when, as a family doctor, I discovered that medical protocols were considered far more important than the actual needs of patients and that my work as a doctor was constantly being monitored by institutions. Was I prescribing enough drugs? Were they the right, the recommended, drugs? Was I following the instructions of specialist doctors? None of this had anything to do with the health of my patients, nor had any of them complained about my work habits or ethics. In fact, I was working as a private doctor in a place where there was no state health system and so patients were free to choose the doctor they wanted.

At first, I thought the problem was inherent within the structure of medicine itself, how it was organised and how it was applied to patients. But in trying to solve the health problems in which the medical profession had lost interest ("hopeless" cases!), I became aware that the problem was actually much larger. The real problem lies at the very foundations of our approach to illness.

In my search for other approaches, I found ways of improving health no one had ever told me about, neither in medical school nor elsewhere. I was surprised to discover that the medical profession was only interested in what they believed to be true, even when they could see with their own eyes that something was not right. The consequence of sharing my new knowledge and interests was professional harassment. The medical authorities, informed about my unusual actions and treatments, ended up threatening me with expulsion. It was then that I knew with certainty that something sinister was lurking deep within the medical establishment.

In time I freed myself from their control by forcing them (it turned out they do not let you go even if you want to) to remove my name from the register of doctors in Britain and renouncing the practice of medicine forever. I began to devote my time to studying health and disease, which quickly became the study of life itself. I realised that science was more than proving you are right, which is what the medical industry does. Science is observing nature, observing what happens when we don't intervene. Science includes all observations, even those that seem strange or unbelievable. Science is sets of theories, not absolute truths, and behind every theory there remain other possibilities until that theory is proven right or wrong. I found that physics and life form the basis of any knowledge about health and disease. By focusing on health rather than on what we think makes us sick, it turns out that disease is easy to understand – once the basic structure of life is understood.

Life is a movement of energy. The entire universe is a bubble of energy, and some of that energy manifests as matter. The type of matter and the way matter behaves, lives and changes over time, is a direct expression of the energy field that has created and is constantly recreating matter. This means that in order to fully understand disease we need to understand the structure of life.

In this book we link the energy of life with the manifestations of life, health and disease. The point of the book is to provide a basic outline to help people understand *how* we become ill. At the same time, hopefully, some will be encouraged to broaden their vision and question the framework of their own knowledge. "Think outside the box" is the signpost to follow.

FOREWORD

Alícia Ninou

This is a book-interview or an interview in book form, whichever you prefer. It has been worked upon during one of the most convulsive times, in terms of health, ever seen. We began the journey in October 2019, only to experience the COVID crisis in March 2020, with the corresponding lockdowns and curfews that were later declared unconstitutional. We ended it in December 2021, when a large part of the population were in full vaccination psychosis and being inoculated with the third dose, on the way to the fourth. We do not know how many more doses may have reached the world's population by the time this book reaches your hands. If by now our contemporaries have not realised what lies behind this sequence of unprecedented events, there is little that can be done to save the common sense of humankind.

This book, free of "viruses" and doses of any kind, is a victory of human insight, a new dawn for a suggested vision and a new understanding of health. Perhaps this is the last chance for those who continue to insist that the enemy is stalking us. No, my friends, the enemy is not out there.

My delightful task has been to decide the issues, to ask the questions, to understand the answers and to ask new questions in order to weave the texts into a coherent and interesting series of chapters. The resulting content has nothing to do with a standard Health Manual, but rather with a philosophical-energetic treatise on self-knowledge and personal self-responsibility. It is a compendium of wisdom that Patrick has compiled from the medicine and ancestral knowledge of Ayurveda, one that has opened my eyes to what really matters, knowledge itself. Ancient civilisations knew this when they said: "Know yourself and you will know the world and the stars."

The thesis of this book is that health is a balance based on self-knowledge. At a time when a plague of covidiots are trying to convince us that there is a virus threatening us all, I would like to vindicate the individuality of health found in these pages. Health, as I see it, is not a social or public issue. We can have all the comforts of the health system and be profoundly and radically ill. Or we can have never visited the doctor and be splendidly healthy. Health is a natural born gift, and is made up of many facets, corners and diagonals that each one of us must deal with in our daily lives. When there is something wrong with us, we should not go knocking at the hospital door, but find our own doors.

What kind of content can you expect here? The proof of the existence of systems in the organism that have nothing to do with the systems that appear in books on medical science or anatomy, as well as the important influence that our expectations play in all processes of life, the brilliance of the energetic organisation of the human body (so many light years away from all that emerges from official knowledge), the real and deep cause of all the processes we call disease, and the deep meaning of the word health.

As for me, I define myself as a freelance journalist. I have been publishing my audiovisual interviews on the website *TimeForTruth. es* and on Youtube and Vimeo. Over the years, I have specialised in giving voice to dissident scientific research and the theories of doctors and professionals working to bring to light different forms of human contamination and intoxication. These include iatrogenics, electromagnetism, chemical contamination, geoengineering and transgenics. My YouTube and Vimeo channels were censored and removed from the network in 2020, with more than 600 videos on them, as a result of the Covidian events we all experienced, and which have degenerated into a health dictatorship.

For some reason I am driven by the search for truth. I could not dedicate myself to anything else. So many years of interviewing people who think outside the box have led me to realise for myself that nothing is what it seems, and that real knowledge has been hidden for centuries for the benefit of a few. Shedding light on small portions of truth is what really moves me.

I cannot end this introduction without mentioning those who made it possible for me to meet Patrick Quanten. My eternal thanks to the SeryActuar team, who discovered his work and started to translate and disseminate it on their website. In 2018, when Patrick came to Spain for the first time, they did not hesitate to propose that I interview him, so I had the pleasure of meeting him in person and the luxury of interviewing him. Secondly, I would like to thank Pilar Aznar, an unconditional friend, for reviewing my translations of Patrick's texts and for her brilliant contributions to the final text, even when she had to give in to some grammatical rebelliousness on my part and to certain literary licences I allowed myself in the final text. Thirdly, to the whole team of the Plural 21 Association, who had the audacity to organise a memorable course with Patrick in Barcelona in October 2019. It was published on my Youtube Channel, which was censored in its entirety in October 2020. You can now enjoy the whole course on the Odysee platform. Finally, my thanks go to the editor, Josep Maria Orteu, who travelled to the town of Balaguer where Patrick participated in the 2019 Food and Health Fair. This was the last one held to date due to the Covid dystopia. He met Patrick personally and proposed the writing of this book-interview on health.

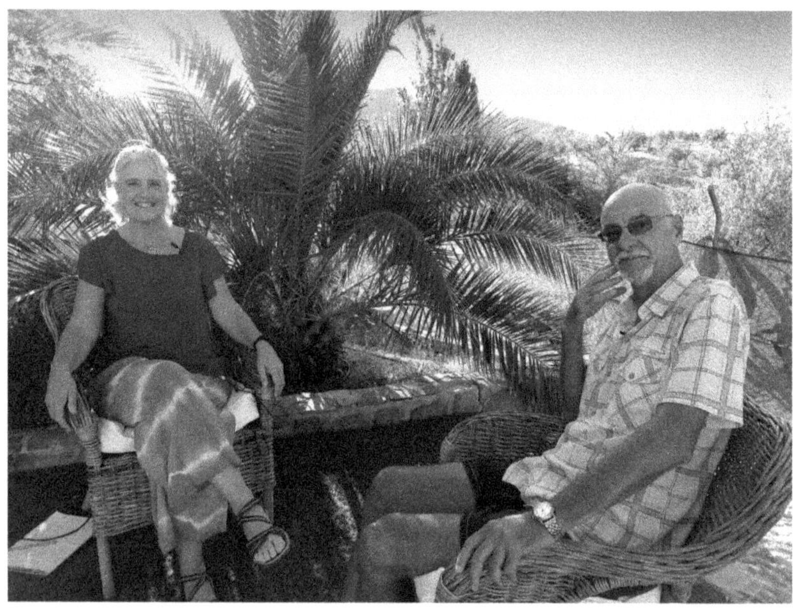

Many of you are probably wondering at this point who Patrick Quanten is. Where did he come from, this doctor who had the courage to give up his professional career to dedicate himself to researching what was never explained to him at university? What is his story? What secrets does he hide? Don't torture yourself. In the next chapter I have prepared a "who's who", a biography of this quixotic and endearing character who, with infinite patience, has answered my questions time and time again until he has hit the bull's eyes.

PATRICK QUANTEN

Patrick was born and raised in Belgium, where he graduated as a medical doctor in 1983. After graduating, he left his home country to start his healthcare career in Great Britain, in a medical practice owned by an elderly doctor on Alderney, a small island off the French coast in the English Channel. After four years of working and learning, the old doctor was unable to carry on working, leaving Patrick as the sole doctor in charge of the practice. This also meant, on such a small island, being available for emergencies 24 hours a day, 7 days a week, and dealing with all kinds of emergencies, varying from family disputes, traffic accidents, cliff accidents, heart attacks and epileptic fits. That was his life for another 14 years, during which time his vision and his appreciation of the medicine he had studied at the university changed gradually and radically.

Practising medicine in such a way was exceptional, not only because of the disparity between and variety of the presenting symptoms, but also because it was private medicine, meaning people had to pay for each consultation, for every service they received and for all the medicines they took. Of course, people like to see results when they are spending their money. On the other hand, living in a small community means that health problems are discussed with the doctor, but not exclusively in the doctor's office. In the bar, the shop, on the street, everywhere people meet they share this information. Random people would ask for information about a patient, of which, as it very often turned out, they knew more than the doctor himself.

It was in this way, crossing paths with his patients in the community, that Patrick soon realised how unsuccessful his medical treatments were. He wondered what the problem was. Did he make mistakes about medical treatments or were they not as effective as they were made out to be? When he referred his patients to medical specialists, for which they had to travel to another island, he noted that the success rate in resolving the health problems of his patients did not improve significantly. In fact, in some cases, the specialist approaches were seriously worsening the situation. But the so say experts never took responsibility. On the contrary, they clung to the belief that the treatments worked, and that, if they didn't, it was the patient's fault, not the medicine. They put this to rest by saying that patients did not follow instructions, did not take their medication or did not realise they were getting better. Patrick knew them all. They were his neighbours, his friends. He knew their lives and their miseries. He continued to observe and, above all, to talk with his patients.

As he was prepared to listen, many of them told him about other therapies such as aromatherapy, chiropractic, osteopathy and reflexology that were unknown to him at the time. He was surprised that these alternative treatments seemed to be working for all kinds of ailments, unlike the medicine that he had been taught, which had very specific diagnoses and protocols. He thought it couldn't be possible, but even so, before discarding the whole idea, he began to study and, over time, he began using these different methods in his own practice.

In this way he began to develop a wide range of therapeutic skills which he practised on his patients, first for those who were interested and later whenever he thought it might be beneficial. Having learned a wide variety of healing skills, he soon had to admit that these different treatments and approaches did not make a real improvement in his success rates. As with official, allopathic, medicine, the other therapies were working for some people, but not for all. They worked some of the time but not every time. The only sensible explanation he could see in all this was that the real cause of the illnesses must have been completely missed, if it had ever been known at all. He also realised another important factor. A therapy, whatever it was, had to be directed at the individual, not at a group.

From that moment on, the search for the true causes of illness became his leading motive in life. First of all, it made him focus his attention on the process of life itself. What is life? How is it structured? Almost without realising it, he found himself studying health rather than investigating disease, discovering that health was related to disease, discovering that health was related to many more aspects of life than he had been shown at university. Where could he learn about life? Many of the answers he found in the major traditions or cosmologies of the millennia of human history. He immersed himself in Traditional Chinese Medicine and in Ayurveda, a medical and philosophical system ten thousand years old. In Ayurveda, he was particularly struck by the fact that it does not treat all people in the same way, but divides them into different groups with similar characteristics in order to better understand the individual symptoms. For example, into "cold" people and "hot" people. Each person then has a unique set of characteristics from several different groups of signs and symptoms. He also became familiar with the energies and the way they shape and move our physical life, and that included the most modern way of investigating energies, quantum physics. Little by little, it all started to make sense in his head. He started to leave behind the doctrine that everything is physical and chemical, and he stood firm in his search for answers in the non-material realm, while continuing to check that what he thought or discovered did not violate the basic principles of life. He moved further and further away from the need to use tools, protocols or drugs to achieve his goal. His goal had now become moving people towards developing their own health. This shift in his practice led to the arrival of some letters from the British Medical Association who were not liking his way of practising medicine. He was not issuing enough prescriptions for someone in his position.

These letters, if anything, opened his eyes even wider to the motives behind Western medicine, to which he was still "tied" through his medical licence. Finally, he decided to cut his ties with the medical profession, as well as with many of his former belief systems. In 2001, Patrick officially relinquished his medical licence, which was not as easy as it might seem. He needed the intervention of a lawyer to get the British General Medical Council to finally remove his name from the General Register of Physicians in England. He learned that the medical profession wasn't an organisation one could simply unsubscribe from when one wished to do so. At that time, among other things, he decided that whatever he was going to do from then on, he would not give it a name, so that he could not be pigeonholed or associated with any group, medicine or therapy ever again. It would become a flight in complete freedom.

After leaving medical practice, he stayed for a few more years on the island of Alderney where he worked as a waiter a couple of days a week. In addition, he continued to see some of his former patients for deep tissue massage, one of the new techniques that he learned and with which he had got some decent results. When he finally left Alderney in 2005, he started to divide his time between England, where his daughter and friends were, and Belgium, with the rest of his family. He opened a private clinic in Belgium with treatments based on Thai massage, the teachings of Buddhism and quantum physics. Once a month he also went to a village in Britain where he gave clinical training and treated and guided individuals towards better health.

In 2007, Patrick published his first book *A Miracle Baby*, in which he tells the story of his daughter's first pregnancy. Early in the pregnancy, the family was informed that the child was not developing properly. Diagnostic tests showed a baby with shrunken kidneys and lungs only partially developing. Statistically speaking, these babies usually die around the sixth month of pregnancy, and Kennedy, that was his name, also looked as if she was heading that way. Regardless, Kennedy's mother, decided that a baby was a baby, and she was going to want it. She was going to love him no matter what his physical condition would be and no matter how long he was going to be with them. She decided that no more scans or ultrasounds to get information or to monitor the process were needed. She simply let herself be guided by how she and the baby felt. Kennedy was born alive on 14 November 2006. He lived for two hours and died in his father's arms.

His next book, in 2017, was *Why Me? Science and Spirituality as inevitable bed partners*, written together with Erik Bualda. It is a scientific study of the human energy field in relation to the energies of evolution, health and disease. It identifies the seven basic frequencies of material creation and shows how the energies passed from one frequency to the next, producing the part of the material world we know now. There is a logical progression in all evolution, which can be followed through the changing energetic field of our universe. At the same time, the book identifies what it means, energetically speaking, when the organism falls ill. In the same way that all material creation stems from pressure that is exerted in the energy field, the logical deduction is that the state in which matter finds itself, whether healthy or diseased, also stems from pressure within the energy field itself. Not only do we know with certainty that life and health/disease are energetic issues, but we can also begin to identify exactly what energetic frequency is causing a problem and where in the energy field that imbalance is located.

Other aspects of Patrick's literary and informational activity can be seen on his websites www.activehealthcare.co.uk and www.pqliar.net. In 2022 he added his new website www.quantics.org in three languages. This is about freedom of belief, how to establish a new faith to help liberate people from the current oppression and slavery of all current governmental systems.

He continues to advance on the path of learning the truths that science has uncovered. By confronting his ideas with real life situations in which individuals find themselves, he has been defining increasingly more precise theories on the origin of diseases and on how to prevent or rectify them. His inside knowledge of allopathic medicine has allowed him to discover where, how and why the truth has been lost, as well as the massive effort that is continually made to not include scientific knowledge in practising medicine, so that medicine can stubbornly adhere to the needs of the industry that has been created, instead of moving towards healing people.

"There is truth in everything", but that also means there is falsehood in everything. Failure to separate the truth from the untruths makes us cling to an *everything*. Clinging to a *whole* will never provide us with the true answers because truth and falsehood remain mixed in the same soup. It is crucial that people keep tracing all observations until they arrive at the basic scientific knowledge that identifies the most obvious falsehoods. There are not many truths in science since everything is theories that are supposed to provide explanations for the observations we make in life. Theories are possible explanations, which means that everything else is still possible too. Patrick's personal journey into science is based on observations related to people's health, and, unlike allopathic medicine, his explanations are based on scientific truth along with related reasoning and justification. Understanding life and the path to health is no longer a mystery to those who really want to understand it.

In 2020, Patrick moved to the south of Spain and retired from his clinical work. He now devotes himself fully to educating people to become self-sufficient and to take full responsibility for their own health. He argues that individuals need to become independent from many things before they will be able to sustain a life separate from existing society. The three main issues he works on are: health, finance and power. His endeavour is to raise awareness about how to build a society without money or any kind of barter system, one free of all forms of debt.

Another thing that occupies Patrick's time is, together with his friend Erik Bualda, co-author of the book *"Why Me?"*, accessing energy that can convert some of the energy of the field in which we live into electricity. This should lead to a completely free and independent energy supply for all individuals. He writes:

> *My own life has always led me to become more and more independent and I am grateful for the opportunity of all those experiences, even though on many occasions I have felt that it was unfair that my life never stabilised, that it kept getting messed up. I kept sabotaging it. My father once said about me: "Why make it easy when you can make it hard on yourself?"*

> *I don't have a dream for my life. I don't have a dream for others or for society. It will be up to each individual to make the most of his or her life. I can only inform and instruct those who are willing to listen, but I do not have any specific goal. I will continue to do what I do, which is being myself, even if no one ever believes a word I say or comprehends*

any action I take. Maybe it won't be now, maybe it's not the moment, but I am sure the moment will come, and I know I could not have done anything other than what I have been doing. I will continue to do it. It was all meant to be and Spain, for now, is the last station of my life's journey. What happens next will be tomorrow's history.

I

WHAT IS HEALTH?

Well, Patrick, since we've set out to talk about health, how about we cut to the chase? Let's begin with the question of what in fact health is.

➤ Health is balance. It's the balance between all influences that affect parts of a system and the balance between all parts of one system.

It is about a balance in energies, the energies that make up all parts of the system. Energies are changed by a change of temperature in the environment and/or a change of pressure in the field, which shows itself as a change of pressure in the tissues (the matter that is the physical result of lowering the pressure in the energy field). Maybe we should add that this balance will change from moment to moment, which means that there is no right way to maintain balance, to be healthy. At the same time, one person's balance will be different from another person's, which shows that there is no general right way to maintain balance, to be healthy.

You consider the human body to be a system? What kind of a system?

➤ The human system begins with the human energy field, that particular part of the universal field that will produce physical humans. This energy field is a further condensation from the mammal field. The human system is, like all other living entities, an ecosystem in itself. Everything in it is always balanced in the sense that all parts move together. The human ecosystem is also part of the universal ecosystem, as it is always in balance with its environment. Everything moves together.

There are seven basic energy frequencies making up this field that will accumulate and condense into a cellular form that contains seven physical systems, each relating to one particular frequency. These are the lymphatic system, circulatory system, breathing/digestive system, motility system, sensory system, nervous system and glandular system. Each of these systems develop into organs. Each organ contains all energies and their manifestations but in different amounts (according to the "Creation Code"). All cells are connected and form the separate organs, and all organs are connected to form the individual.

The human field contains the energies for manifesting all physical human beings. Every human being is made up of a structure that holds the organs, and the organs are made up of cells. Hence the human system consists of an energy field and a physical aspect. The physical aspect is made up of cells that form organs and it all functions as a unit, as one system.

The Creation Code

What do you mean when you talk about the "Creation Code"?

☙ Creation is a continuous manifestation of condensed energies. This happens on a repetitive basis, meaning that the same things happen over and over again. Wherever we look within the universe we should always find the same system of manifestation. This can then be expressed in a single code which represents the pattern used by the universe on its journey of manifestation. That code we have discovered, so we now know how the universe developed, is developing and how it is going to develop further.

It is tempting to talk about the universe, but let's not forget that this is a book about health, so let's go back, for now, to what you call the "condensed human system". What must we humans do to maintain balance in our system, so that we don't get sick?

☙ The two main concepts about the balance of a system are, firstly, that balance is personal and non-transferable, and secondly, that balance will be constantly changing. This makes it obvious that there is no advice that can be given to anyone about what is the healthiest lifestyle or the healthiest diet for them. It all depends on the individual.

But there is another important factor in this dynamic, and that is that life has always found a way to move on, to find its balance. Nature is always in balance, whatever circumstances or forces are at work at any given moment. Without our help, without our interference, life is always in balance. In other words, we don't really need to do anything to keep ourselves healthy and balanced. But if we intend to interfere directly and choose to be part of our balancing act, we would do well first to understand what happens in our bodies and how our nature responds to changing influences.

We need to learn about life and, in particular, about our own life. There are general laws to be considered in nature, laws that will be enacted even when we are doing our best to alter the course of events. A simple example of this is that we are all going to grow old, become decrepit and die, no matter what we do to try to alter that chain of events, that natural biological process. If we truly want to contribute to maintaining the balance of our systems rather than trying to randomly alter them, there are two steps to take:

1. To learn about balance in our own life

2. To learn how we can more easily maintain that balance

Basic principles of nature

Let's talk about those general laws of nature that we cannot alter. We are all supposed to know them, aren't we?

-● Maybe it is better to call them universal principles instead of laws. Here they are:

- All life has a beginning, an expansion stage, a contraction stage and an end.

- Everything has an influence on everything else through an exchange of energies, one thing responding to another.
- Nothing is created out of nothing.
- The seed is already present and responding to its environment, to incoming information.
- What goes up must come down. There is a limit to the response before it will turn back on itself. An expansion can only go so far before it begins to contract again.
- Life is movement and it moves in circles.
- Life is cyclical, never reaching the same point again as that point also moves on.
- The true movement is a spiral.
- Life is an entwining of spirals.

As we will go along, we might come across other general universal truths but for now this is a starting point.

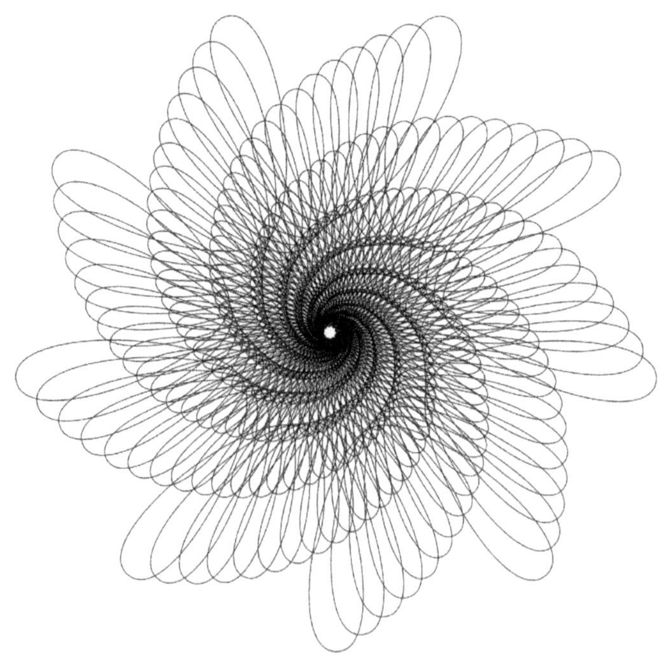

In the midst of so much change, up and down, circles, spirals, it seems a bit difficult to maintain the vital balance you are talking about. What would be the rules for maintaining it?

We can't change circles and spirals, so we don't need to put any energy into that. Furthermore, we don't even need to know the circles and spirals themselves. All we need to concern ourselves with is the effect those influences have on individuals.

We need to understand that any circumstance in itself is neither good nor bad. When it is raining does that mean it is bad weather? That all depends on your point of view, on your particular needs. When you are born in a very challenging environment does that make for a good or a bad life? That depends on the kind of personality you are born with and on what happens next. Whether something is going to have a supportive or a destructive influence on a person, keeping him healthy or making him ill, will depend on how he responds to influences.

Virtually all of our lives are being lived unconsciously. We are not aware of what needs to happen when we eat an apple. If life is an unconscious affair, how can we know whether something is a good or a bad influence on us? Our tiny consciousness does not receive any messages from the unconscious routines of living, as long as there is nothing wrong. When something out of the ordinary happens, we get a signal. These are general indications such as a headache, feeling nauseous, shoulder pain, being unable to sleep, fever and skin eruptions. These signals are usually short lived, disappearing quickly of their own accord. What does this mean? Two things:

1. The system has momentarily been pushed out of balance.
2. The system has rectified the imbalance on its own.

Recurrent signals indicate that there is potentially an underlying problem whereby small alterations in the environment result in a momentary imbalance of the system. It means that at that point the system does not have much reserve, much flexibility.

From this we can see that the first part of maintaining a balance is to learn about ourselves. We need to learn how to read the signs and signals our bodies (and minds) are giving us. In order for us to be able to observe what the system does to try and restore the balance, we need to learn not to interfere quickly. Only by waiting can we learn this part. We need to learn who we are, how we are structured and what our weak and our strong points are. It is only by knowing ourselves in a deeper sense that we can make sense of the signals our consciousnesses are receiving.

If everything depends on responses to influences, and in each person the responses are different, then a diagnosis cannot be made on the basis of symptoms. The same symptoms can mean different things to different people. This means there is no such thing as a diagnosis and there is no such thing as a disease, doesn't it?

Indeed. There are no general diagnoses because a signal can mean different things to different people and different things at different times.

The signals, physical signs as well as emotional and mental states, are like words in a language. They can mean different things in different circumstances. And, just as in a language where you have many dialects with the same sounding words meaning different things, the same signals in different people may also mean something different. The thing to remember is that you only need to be able to communicate with your own system. It is the only system you have any responsibility for. We all need to learn to listen to our own signs.

How can this be done? We have to learn a new language. We listen to the sounds, the intonations, to find out what the mood of the "talking" is. We try to feel whether the signal relates to high tension or lack of tension. What does it feel like? How would you describe the signal, the sign? Like a tight band around the head? Like light-headiness? Pressure on the eyes? A bloated stomach? Weakness in the voice? Muscle cramps? Describe what it feels like. Very often the answer to the first question regarding the meaning of the signal is already there.

When we receive a high tension signal via the tissues it means that there must be high tension in the energy field, on a non-material level, on a mental or emotional level, too, so now we want to know when this occurs. For this we need to observe the signal but at the same time also the circumstances in which it shows up. I am talking about the energetic circumstances, the atmosphere in which the sign occurs.

Regarding signs, can you give me some practical examples?

🍂 Of course. Let's look at a couple of them:

Painful cramping in the tummy with headaches and feeling sick, always before menstruation. Ask yourself: "What am I holding on to? What is so difficult to let go of? What have I, as a woman, against menstruating?"

Feeling sick with tummy cramps and occasional diarrhoea.

What has gone before? Is it when I am tired? Stressed? Worried? Afraid? Overrun with questions I can't answer? Working against a deadline?

It is never the tomato or the chocolate or the coffee. Try and look at the mental state in which the signal occurs.

Observing over and over again will provide you with more and more detailed information which will eventually allow you to come up with a theory about the background to the signal. Now you have an idea as to why this may be occurring. You need to have an understanding about what is going on before you should interfere. When you interfere you need to know how you mean to influence the situation and what effect that would have. Then you can observe the reality and use that as feedback towards your initial theory.

Right. If I find I get a tummy ache and diarrhoea when I'm stressed, do I try not to get stressed the next time? Or if I find I'm tired, do I try not to get so tired? Or if I have a fight with my husband, do I try to make up? You mean we should never act directly against the signal, but according to its meaning?

-☙ Indeed, your interference should start with the signal and your understanding of it. However, when you keep observing your understanding may deepen and what first looked like a direct link between a stressful situation and the physical sign may, after some reoccurrences, tell you that there is more going on.

The universal principle that says that everything is interconnected leads to a very specific conclusion when one keeps observing signals and signs. This is that there is never just one reason behind the signal. The signal indicates an acute imbalance between the inner world and the outer world. Hence when trying to figure out what the meaning of a signal is one should always look on the outside and always on the inside. For example, if I am currently in a stressful situation that may well be a powerful influence, but the question that should also be asked is: "why am I responding this way right now?"

You may find yourself in a stressful situation for a few weeks, or years, and then I would be interested to know why you had a tummy upset only yesterday. What was the additional factor that made the signal appear? This is the crucial point for beginning the healing process. You need to know what made you respond in that particular way at that particular time. Why? Because most of the time you will be unable to change outside influences as they are out of your control (weather, pressure of work, disasters, accidents, etc.) but you do have the power to change the inside responses.

You can only effectively begin to heal when you understand why and how you respond to certain circumstances.

The relative importance of food

You mentioned that food is not related to health. I find it strange that you say that. Would you like to clarify?

-☙ Food is an exchange of information. We use food to give us more information about our surroundings and the state they are in. Food brings us information about the abundance of life or scarcity of life. It lets the inner world know whether or not the outside world has a lot to offer or not. So, it brings information about the climate, about the seasons, about the weather conditions, about the quality of the soil and water. When this information corresponds with information our system receives from other sources such as vision, sounds and smells, it allows it to make definite adjustments for living under those outside conditions. When we eat food that does not belong to the season, does not belong in this climate or does not rot, the system gets confusing messages and its response to our environment will be torn between opposing possibilities. Inside there will be doubt and whatever the system does it won't be the best it could do. as some things are forcing it to hold back.

The ingredients in what we eat do not have to comply with a list of how much we need of every single molecule. The ingredients of oranges reflect this year's ripening season and so they should be different from last year's. When, in general terms, a specific crop fails one year there is a natural reason for that and that reason also shows itself in other aspects of life. For our systems it is then best that we do not have that food item this year, because that information coincides with what the system has picked up elsewhere and will therefore enforce the message of failure, of disaster. Eating natural foods within their seasons will always bring balanced messages to the system. Therefore, there is no direct link between what we eat and our diseases, but food can bring a message of despair or pending death. In that case it isn't the poor quality of food that will kill us or make us ill but the reason for the scarcity of food or the lack of quality that will affect us. And when nature is dying all around us our lives become threatened too.

Please clarify further. There are many medical systems that rely on food as a method of healing, for example, naturopathy, hygienism and Ayurveda. There is a philosophy of life that says, "We are what we eat", encouraging us to try to eat as naturally as possible, without additives or toxins, in order to be healthy. I find it hard to believe that there is no direct relationship between our food and

our health. Isn't it important to take care over our food? It is our body's fuel, so shouldn't it be the best possible fuel?

-🝔 This is a mistake. The body's primary fuel is oxygen. We have two integrated systems to fuel our activities: digestion and breathing. These systems exist in every cell, and through them the cellular organism can turn solid material and gases into fuel. The use of gases to extract the necessary fuel substances is much easier than the same process with solids. "Easier" means it costs less energy: the energy investment for extraction is far less in gases than in solids. This is no different from human beings extracting energy sources from the earth. It takes a lot more energy to get coal then it does to extract oil or gas.

The other important point is that the cells use the solids they have access to in their immediate environment whenever they are asked to produce energy from solid material. The cell's environment is the inner working of our system. What materials are available in the extracellular space? The matter that is contained in the stomach is a very long way away from that extracellular environment.

Can we find scientific proof for this theory?

-🝔 Indeed we can. The food that we eat ends up in the stomach and will be absorbed during its passage through the gut. Broken down food items (smaller molecules) will be moved by the cells of the lining of the gut into the blood stream. The venous blood that takes away what the cells eliminate will take it straight to the liver. The entire circulatory system of the stomach and gut is separate from the larger circulatory system that supplies the rest of the body. The hepatic circulatory system runs directly from the cells of the gut to the liver. In the liver the blood vessels open up into large spaces where the liver cleans up all the contents. It breaks down the molecules and recycles the small molecules and atoms. The liver is the largest internal detoxification organ we have. Everything that is absorbed into the hepatic circulatory system has to pass through the liver first before the blood continues its journey to the lungs, to pick up energy (from oxygen) – and from there to the cells of the body.

Furthermore, life is energy, not matter. Life functions as an energetic system: it doesn't require matter to function. The exchanges in life are energetic exchanges. So vibrational messages are being passed from one system to another or from one environment to another. We eat to internalise messages from our environment. The messages are encoded within matter and once the message has been received the matter has done its job and becomes redundant. It will be broken down and eliminated immediately.

A health system built on matter exchanges and matter interactions is never going to give you effective answers to questions about health and is never going to contribute to balancing life. However, once you have constructed such a system and you have invested in such a system you are likely to do anything you can to make it grow. You will emphasise every small possible connection you can find. You have to expose people to nothing else but your idea that matter is what life is all about, so you put all the material bits at the centre of your policy: exercise, food, CO_2 in the air and so on.

The petrochemical industry owns the pharmaceutical industry, and they own the food industry, and they own the supplement and herbal products industry. Why would they advise you of anything else?

When Ayurveda became known in the West, food was put forward as the most important item. Traditionally, the hierarchy is somewhat different. Foremost, there is the state of the mind (meditation is the most important tool), followed by breathing, then the physical asanas (positions for opening up the physical channels) and lastly there is food.

Physical exercise

I understand, food is a part of health – we have to eat – but not an important part. On the other hand, you also mentioned exercise as something material. Isn't walking, running, playing a sport or stretching important to health either?

➜ Exercise is a modern invention to exploit people who don't move.

Human beings are constructed so they can move. We are supposed to move and have always moved, but each individual has been constituted for a different purpose. A violinist has been built differently from a high jumper. Together with talent, a person has a body structure to allow that talent to be expressed. Through the expression of that talent the body will get trained in that particular direction. The seamstress is able to manage the specific strains of the job, as is the cobbler or the gondolier in Venice. Each of those people moves through the day with purpose and is made for the strain of those particular movements. He or she will suffer little in comparison to anyone else occasionally trying to do the same job. From a natural health point of view there are two important points to remember here:

- A person's physical body should be stressed by movements he/she was made for.
- A person should move with a purpose, with the goal to achieve something specific.

When we are building the framework of our life it should be based on the strong parts of our constitution. What we are good at should be emphasised and trained. It is not a good idea to have a job or career because there are lots of opportunities in that direction. It should be because you are made for it. It is the relevant parts of the whole system and the physical body that you should train mostly.

Any exercise programme – and that includes yoga when it is used simply as a way of exercising – has no specific purpose in nature. It is a compensation for not moving and for not having a purpose for moving. Sadly, you can't compensate for the lack of something. If you want your life to become better, you will have to discontinue not having a purpose for moving. Not moving, or not having to move, cannot be compensated for by moving strenuously without a purpose. It only eats up even more energy.

Ah, so it burns calories and that must be good for you, especially when you are otherwise not moving much?

-🠖 Sadly, energy levels and energy flow cannot be measured in terms of calories. Physics has long ago abandoned the machine model. We do not function like machines. We are energetic beings wherein the flow of energy and the level of flow will be determined by lots and lots of influences, not simply the balance of intake and burning of calories.

Not everybody is made to run and those who are can easily be divided into fast runners for short distances and slower runners for longer distances. They are clearly constituted differently. Not everybody is made for doing physical sports. However, everybody is made to walk, to twist, turn and bend. We should be using the movements the body has been made for and on top of that we should be training the movements we need to get better at whatever purposes we have.

Health is a balance, and the movement of the individual should be in balance with his or her daily activities. That is the balance within the physical realm but there should also be a balance of mind and body. This means that physical movements should coincide with a mind-set that supports that physical routine. And this unit, mind and body, should be in balance with the natural surroundings of the individual. In other words, one should live in an environment where one's physical capacities are useful assets for survival.

As far as I can see, being healthy in our society must be very complicated. Many of us have very sedentary jobs, with purposes that do not involve physical effort. In my case, I spend all day in front of a computer. Many live in urban environments with few opportunities to walk in nature. When a person in this situation becomes ill, would you recommend a total change of lifestyle?

-🠖 Yes, when anybody, not just a city person, becomes ill, imbalanced, a significant change in life is always required. You mention outside factors as causes of diseases, but the actual disease is an individual reaction to that environment, to those impulses. This means that an imbalanced person must look at how they allow the outside world to impact their individual life. The end result, as the disease state indicates, is imbalance and in order to re-balance that particular life they will need a different framework. They needs to live differently and that involves having different reactions to the impulses, to the outside world.

What about herbs, vitamin supplements, minerals and orthomolecular medicine? Do they serve a beneficial purpose?

⬤ Therapy can never be a cure because the disease is an imbalance between the inner world of the person and their outer world. That balance or imbalance is caused by the reaction of that person to outside stimuli. For such reaction to cause a disease, an imbalance, it needs to be present for a long time. This means we are talking about a reaction pattern. This is an unconscious way of responding to the environment and the impulses that are present in the environment. For this reaction pattern to change we need to understand what the reaction pattern is, and where and how it can be changed. In order to understand, someone needs to observe constantly. To alter a pattern, they need to constantly monitor and adjust. Both of these tasks can only be carried out by being in the present all the time and with the capability of adjusting at any given moment. This can only be done by the person concerned, not by an outsider.

The outsider, and we can call that person a therapist, can help someone to focus and can provide methods to help him or her to observe better and to make adjustments more efficiently.

Life is energy, so effective adjustments involve altering energies (thoughts, feelings and belief systems). For the pattern to be changed the change in energies must be permanent and it therefore has to come from within someone, from the unconscious governing field that rules their responses.

What kind of help can we expect from therapies and any influence from the outside?

◕ Whenever you alter a routine, the system will have to sit up and take notice. It will receive a wake-up call. The system will then evaluate the inner situation and begin to adjust. For example, when you start to take vitamin supplements every day, the system becomes more alert and begins to rectify whatever has been slowly going wrong. Hence the initial positive effect on your wellbeing. When you begin smoking cannabis daily, you will begin to feel better, whatever your initial complaints were. When you begin drinking 2 litres of water every day you will start to feel much better pretty quickly. But that also happens when you start to drink coffee or alcohol, or you start eating dhal! The same thing happens when you stop doing things you had been doing regularly. When you remove food items from your diet you will begin to feel better very quickly. Anything you take or you leave out will give you a better feeling. That is caused by the change you have made. It has forced the system to not simply respond, almost blindly, to the daily routine but to now "think" about it. It has to construct a new, different, responsive pattern.

Initially that can result in a partial rectification of imbalances. However, the system is always looking to convert responses into patterns. Responding unconsciously, without any thought, evaluation or consideration, costs a lot less energy than constantly having to make decisions on how and what. Think about how difficult it is to learn to ride a bike. How much effort and concentration it requires. Then, after some time, it becomes natural. You ride the bike automatically. It has become a habitual pattern that deals, unconsciously, with all aspects of riding a bike.

When the system has been shocked by altering a routine and this has caused a significant effect, this effect is described as positive because the system has been forced to re-evaluate and to respond differently. This results in rectifying existing imbalances. Now that you are carrying out this new routine, because it does you "good", the system will soon adjust the unconscious pathways to incorporate your new routine. From then on, the system goes to sleep again and continues its deeper response patterns, incorporating the new one without allowing it to throw the system off course. The positive shock effect disappears and the old existing routine responses surface once again.

The results of this are seen in all helping and caring professions. For example, doctors notice that after some time they frequently have to increase the strength of the medication in order to establish an effect. Where years ago, you only needed to go and see the osteopath twice a year, now you need to visit him every month. Where drinking this herbal tea cured my recurrent cystitis some years back, I now have all the symptoms back again. Where using a walking stick initially gave me more stability, and I was certainly walking better, it now no longer provides me with a feeling of security and my walking is deteriorating even further.

> For all of this there is just one reason. All those interventions have not affected the cause of the disease, the cause of the original imbalance. The cause of a disease is the fundamental response pattern from one organism to the world it lives in. All we do with these interventions is to force the system to change the surface, not the deeper roots of the responses.

What does that mean? Have a look at which interference suggestions someone wants to try and which he rejects. Ask yourself why someone is willing to drink a particular herbal tea but is not willing to meditate twice a day because that would disturb their existing routine. Now begin to pay more attention to what someone rejects rather than what they is willing to try. Soon you will find out that the changes the person rejects or abandons quickly are the ones that would make a much deeper impact on the routine automatic unconscious responses that person uses. It is these changes that come a lot closer to altering the response pattern at a deeper level, therefore potentially curing the person of the imbalance he or she experiences right now.

People want to have a better life, with less pain, stress and pressure, but they are not willing to give up what they have known all their lives. The fear of changing what we already know, what makes us feel safe and secure, is far greater than our need to find harmony. There is a belief that harmony must come from the outside world: "if only others would be kind and help me, life would be so much better", "if only others wouldn't cheat so much, I would have less stress". In essence, this is clinging to what you want instead of living based on what is there corresponds to an unconscious pattern of response that ends up becoming a prison.

Could you give an example of this please? It seems important.

➤ It is far more important than it looks. We can illustrate this very well by looking at the behaviour of a monkey and be aware that we are just like monkeys. You fix a box to a tree. The box has a hole in it so the monkey can reach inside. Inside the box you place a banana. The monkey finds the box with the banana, puts his hand inside the box, grabs the banana but is unable to get his hand out of the box whilst holding on to the banana. Indigenous people catch monkeys that way. They only need to go up to the box where the monkey is still holding on to the banana and pick him up. In order to escape, all the monkey needs to do is to let go of the banana and then he can run away. But he doesn't!

People do not want to give up what they believe in, what they have known all their life, even if it will heal them. The suggestions they reject with vigour are more than likely to be the ones they need to follow the most. When they do alter these deep-seated responses, their life will change forever.

The signals

I laughed a lot at the story of the monkeys. Although it is really sad, it illustrates the mentality of many people very well. But how guilty are these people? As children, we are not taught how our system works. As adults, unfortunately we don't have the knowledge that you are sharing. Moreover, people don't only receive one

signal at a time. Many people receive a lot of signals at the same time, probably caused by different causes or imbalances. Over the years they accumulate. How do I do this jigsaw puzzle? How do I know which signal corresponds to which cause? Is this where I may need a therapist or a doctor to help me?

♨ We all have a multitude of responses that we unconsciously make from our reaction patterns. The signals we receive from the physical body, and sometimes from the mind (perhaps tiredness, depression or lack of joy), are not as complex and manifold at any given time as we might think.

In order to begin analysing the signals we first have to make a judgement about what needs our attention and might usefully be adjusted. That first judgement is about what signals are important for us to notice. When signals appear and disappear quickly, we take notice and remember, but don't need to do anything about them. When a signal appears, it means that at that moment in time the system is struggling. When it disappears, without us doing anything, it means the system has got it under control. Only when we notice certain signals recurring or signals no longer disappearing, it indicates that the system is not overcoming the pressure problem. Then we should take notice of what we are feeling. Where can I feel the pressure? What exactly am I feeling? How would I describe it in words? There is often a lot of information in the words we use. In addition, we need to take notice of the circumstances in which the signal occurs.

When? How does it occur? What exactly happens?

♨ Until we have enough information to formulate a theory about what is happening to us, we should not take any action, as all action will alter the way the system will respond. This would seriously cloud the information we are seeking.

Once you have established that it isn't the tomato that gives you tummy cramps and diarrhoea, you can ask yourself questions such as: "How am I feeling just before the signal appears? What have I been thinking? What am I worried about? What company have I been in?" Gradually you can discover the real circumstances in which your system begins to complain.

By not doing anything about the reaction the system is having, but instead observing everything that relates to that time and place, you will begin to understand the important links much better. Once you develop a theory about what inside of you is causing the signal you are receiving from your system, it becomes obvious that you need to do the exact opposite to reduce that particular pressure. Then you start doing that and you keep observing the effect of your action, your interference. That will tell you if you are right or not.

So no, you don't need a specialist or a doctor. All you need is patience and to trust that your system is not going to destroy itself. It is trying to tell you something and since the two of you speak a different language, it takes a lot of repeating and gesturing for you to understand the message. Being patient and using a lot of guess work will get you there. Don't forget that you are the only one who can have this kind of conversation with your system. All signals come from one and the same system, yours. That means that all signals tell you something about the main imbalance you are suffering from. All signals relate at some level to each other. Don't separate them: try to join them all up.

As I understand you, the things that can help us to improve are reflection, calmness, observation and meditation.

 Yes, in order to improve our understanding of life and our connection with life we need the following steps, in this order:

1. Gaining theoretical knowledge about how life has been constructed and how in general it functions

2. Observing how that knowledge shows up in your own life

3. Testing the knowledge through observing the effects of interference

4. Learning techniques and methods for intervening in useful ways

What exactly is meditation for you?

-● Meditation can be a lot of things but the most important, the most effective, part is *to live it* rather than to practise it. Meditation is a way of concentrating the mind. Keeping focus does not allow the mind to freely wonder in all kinds of directions. This has two enormous benefits for our life. One is that the mind becomes a lot quieter, more restful, because it is not jumping up and down all the time. And secondly, what we are focussing on will become empowered and will therefore manifest in the most effective and most powerful way. Living with a focussed mind, not becoming distracted by details, sets out direct lines in your life. Then the mind knows what is expected of it and it will carry that out without doubt, without wavering, without fear.

I think these steps or stages you mention are well worth a new chapter, don't you?

-● Sure, why not? How about talking about how life has been constructed and how it works?

What life do you mean, human lives?

-● I mean Life with a capital L. Life in general.

The delusion that the world has not yet come to realise this important truth, and to foresee the harm that follows to the human republic from the indifferent use of physicians, arises principally from three causes:

1. It is considered difficult to know how to medicate oneself, even though we can see that all other animals cure themselves.

2. We take it for granted that doctors have all the knowledge necessary for good medicine. We are certainly mistaken in that. Ordinarily, doctors know less than the sick themselves.

3. Almost everyone makes use of doctors. As we govern ourselves by blindly following the common opinion, the example of others encourages us to follow. As Father Malebranche says: *Ex opinione vivimos, aliorumque exemplum nos facit audaciones.* "We live by the opinion and the example of others, which makes us more audacious".

4. The common example has great persuasion power because it appears to be so much more universal. There is no doubt that this would be the case, if the ignorant were not vastly greater in numbers than the learned men. But to us this seems the very thing that gives it its value and it is also the thing that condemns it: nothing is more suspicious than a great number of approvers, of followers. Truth is not to be found in the number of people believing the statement.

Fragment from the book
Ayer y Hoy. El mundo engañado por los falsos medicos
Miquel Masgrau I Bartis
An address given by Dr. Josef Gazola, medic and academic
Posthumous work
1st edition, *Il mundo ingannato de falsi medici,* Verona, 1716
Bestseller in the eighteenth century

II

HOW DOES LIFE FUNCTION?

You proposed that we talk about the function of life, and here we are. Why do you think this knowledge is necessary for being healthy? Can I be healthy without knowing anything about the functioning of life, or not?

♠ You can, but you won't have any controlling impact if you don't understand it. When you better understand life, how it is constructed and how it functions, you can find ways to contribute more efficiently to the smooth functioning of your life. Look at operating a machine, a car for instance. You can drive your car smoothly and the engine can sound, even be, "healthy". However, if you don't understand the mechanics of the car, you won't know what is wrong, be able to fix any kind of problem or even know what it needs to remain healthy.

All we know about health is what we have been told. All our actions in relation to our health are based on what we know, which is what we have been told. How do you know what you have been told is the truth? Is it worth questioning what you have been told?

♠ Yes, of course! We think we know a lot of things but in reality these are mostly acts of faith. We don't question who is saying it or why. I started questioning when I observed that certain statements were not true. Simple observation convinced me I hadn't been told the truth, or that what I had been told could not be the truth. For example, I was told that smoking caused lung cancer, but I noticed that some people with lung cancer had never smoked and that some people who smoked all their lives did not get lung cancer. What I had been told could not have been the truth. There had to be more to it than that.

Simple observations show you, time and time, again that we are not being told the truth. Once I realised that, in general, I was not being told the truth I began to make more and more conscious observations. Everything is still presented as if all that matters is matter, while a hundred years ago science proved that all, including matter, is energy. So everything about the world I live in, and the way I perceive that world, has been put together back to front. It isn't first matter and then, here and there when it is convenient, energy. Since then I have known that if the explanation I receive is a materialistic one, it can't be the truth. There is more to it than I am being told.

In other words, we live in an upside-down world?

☙ Of course, and it is by observing how things really are, not just believing what we are told, that we can appreciate this.

The great deception

It takes courage to recognise that one has been deceived. When you start to realise this you have to face yourself and others. Can you tell us how and when you discovered the great deception? As a doctor attempting to help people it must have been very difficult.

☙ The key for me was living in a small, isolated community, an island in the English Channel, where you could meet any neighbour at any time, in the bar, in the shop, in the street, practising a hobby, literally anywhere. I knew what they each did for a living, their routines, their likes and dislikes, their passions and their habits.

I left university with a book under my arm, one filled with recipes and prescriptions for curing all kinds of illnesses. For those conditions that could not be cured, there were clear instructions on how to limit the disease's progression, its development and its impact on people's lives.

With that I thought that very soon no one would be sick or suffering unnecessarily on that island. "At last I have come! Your saviour is here!". But the "saviour" in me soon began to be disappointed as I realised that, although I was following what the books said to the letter, many people did not improve in the way they were meant to. First I blamed myself. Then I started to seek help from other professionals with more training and experience than me. I referred patients to different specialists and even brought some of those specialists to the island for private consultations.

Later, as I opened my mind to other possibilities, I started to involve homeopaths and osteopaths as well, but I was still disappointed with the results. I kept having patients who didn't get better. I didn't like that because my medical books did not mention failure. I observed that when specialists were confronted with the failure of their treatment or of their medical advice their usual explanation was to blame the patient: "He's not taking his medication", "He's still secretly drinking or smoking" or "He's imagining it". As I knew these patients, their lives and their habits well, I was often able to defend them and express my disagreement with the specialist. However, the only response I got was disbelief and rejection.

I felt I had no choice but to start looking for alternatives, often encouraged by patients who came to me and asked me if I knew this or that therapy, which I, of course, did not. I began to study, with eagerness and urgency, everything that came my way. I also invited, and paid for, experts to come to the island to give lectures, workshops or simply to instruct me. Unfortunately, I never found what I was looking for, an approach, a treatment that would always work, for everyone.

After studying Traditional Chinese Medicine for a while, I abandoned that in order to study the ancient medical and philosophical system of Ayurveda, Traditional Indian Medicine. Somehow, I understood much better what I read about Ayurvedic science than what I read about conventional Western medicine. Surprisingly, I somehow understood it much better. For the first time in my adult life I began to understand that there was a structure behind life. The only other complete structure I had found before this had been in the scriptures of the Catholic church. I was born into a Catholic community and went to a Catholic school and university. As a teenager I rejected the Catholic teachings and turned away from religion altogether. I dismissed the idea of a pious authority that would judge my life and decide whether I deserved to go to heaven or hell. I rebelled against the idea of punishment and against the belief that I could only fulfil God's designs by believing and adhering to the words of another human being. I could not accept that.

The science of Ayurveda brought me back to the structure of the universe and of life, but this time presented in a more neutral way, not in human terms. I discovered an energetic structure of life, although I must admit that at that time I was not even aware of what that really meant. Energy was something that was not even mentioned in the institutions where I had studied to become a doctor. To my surprise, I discovered that on many occasions what I had been taught in medical school was just the opposite of Ayurvedic teachings. From then on, I began to distance myself from the truth I had been told at university.

Gradually I began to look around me at human beings and the outside world according to what I was learning about in Ayurveda. When I could, I would quietly interpret what I saw around me by trying to place in the framework of Ayurveda. Little by little everything began to make sense. The more I observed, the more free I felt from the ideas imposed by the academic world and the more receptive my mind became to answers coming incessantly from other sources, other places. My natural curiosity was pleasantly stimulated to the point where I felt a real need to free myself from the shackles of my academic profession. Deep down, I knew that staying in the profession could only lead to confrontation. I realised I would not be able to win that battle or to survive it, so I gave up my medical licence and left the profession. I did it mainly to block a thought in the back of my mind. That thought was being voiced to me by my loved ones: "If financial difficulties arise, you can always return to the profession for short periods of time, to cover holiday or sickness leave for other doctors.". I didn't want that to happen, so I decided to sever all links with the medical profession and to force myself to move forward and focus on my new purpose, without looking back and without the safety net of earning money by returning to the profession when needed.

So, your current view of the structure of human life, how it has been built and how it functions, does it come from Ayurveda? What is the structure of life according to this worldview?

➥ Ayurveda is the basis. From that basic structure I started to look further for more conclusive answers. My line of investigation was not to pursue one dogma or another but to stick to a framework and its basic rules. The governing principles I subscribe to are:

- Everything is structured in the same way, so in and out are similar, above and below are similar, front and back are similar.
- There is no loss or gain, only change.
- There are no exceptions in the structure or the function of the universe.
- All serious attempts to explain life that are built on observations have value and should, ultimately, have a place within the true explanation.

Ayurveda says that there is one ever present power in life. It is called Prana, meaning the energy of life. It divides into two forces, a contracting force and an expanding force.

In Chinese philosophy there is life energy, chi, which has yin, contracting, and yang, expanding, effects.

In the Bible there is the ever present power called God, which splits into the Holy Trinity: the Father, the Son and the Holy Ghost.

In quantum physics there is an ever present power, energy (everything is energy), which gives rise to two more fundamental forces of the universe, namely the strong force, which makes things converge onto one another, and the weak force, which makes things part.

In Ayurveda these three forces are said to give rise to 5 elements, out of which everything in creation occurs. These elements indicate a shift from loose, mobile and fast to hard, compact, stabile and slow. They are ether, air, fire, water, earth. Fire relates directly to the power of energy and lies at the centre. The contracting force creates water and later earth. The expanding force creates air and later ether. [1]These five elements give rise to seven tissues that can be found in all living organisms. Every animal, plant and even bacteria has been found to be made out of these seven tissues and structures. The gradation from open, loose and fluid towards compact, solid and fixed, can be identified. Each tissue emerges out of the previous one and is more compact than the one before. They are all interconnected and interdependent. They are represented in terms of bodily tissues and their names refer to some of the major characteristics of the types of tissues and structures they represent. The names given to these tissues are:

- tissue of juices/skin
- tissue of blood
- tissue of muscle
- tissue of fat
- tissue of bone
- tissue of nerve
- tissue of seed

With that framework of universal structure, based on ancient knowledge from across the ages and across the globe, we can now begin the task of trying to fit into it what we observe of creation.

---

[1] Air: the "atmosphere" surrounding a material space object (planet or star). Ether: the "substance" that fills the space in between the material manifestations within the universe.

The first thing that was created in this universe is visible light. "Visible" means it is manifestly present in the universe. It was the very first thing according to the Bible in its first verse: And God said, "Let there be light: and there was light and it became light". Modern scientists talk about an explosion at the very beginning of creation.

And let light now consist of seven colours! Perhaps we need to study the structure of visible light to get an idea of the structure of the entire universe. I admit that I am a bit confused by your introduction to the seven body tissues and the seven colours of light. Where is this leading?

◗ That is understandable. The old Ayurvedic knowledge talks about seven tissues, which I had never heard of before, and modern science tells me that there are seven colours in the first thing that appeared in our universe. If everything is constructed in the same way, could it then be that the formation of the tissues has a relationship with the colours of the visible light?

The golden ratio

Then I come across something else I wasn't told about in school. Apparently throughout human history scientists as well as artists have used a very specific structure to either describe the world around them or to create something in harmony. This principle is used in architecture, paintings, and sculpture, and has been noted in the arrangement of seeds in a sunflower, the places where new branches sprout out of old ones, the shapes of snail shells, and elsewhere. The principle is generally known as the Golden Ratio. It can be expressed in geometric shapes or in a mathematical form. Two consecutive figures are added up to form a third one. Then this one is added to the previous figure to form the next one and so on – 0, 1, 1, 2, 3, 5, 8, 13, 21 etc. So now I wonder whether the Golden Ratio is the way everything in nature is structured and whether that is what we perceive as harmony.

What do we know about the division of the visible light into seven colours?

➤ Each colour has a specific bandwidth, a specific beginning and a specific ending. In between there is a gradual change within the colour[2] as the frequencies[3] move from low to high. Not all colours cover the same widths of frequencies. Some have narrow bands. Others have wider bands.

Why? How are these characteristics being produced?

➤ After a lot of research and puzzling we discovered that the colours within the visible light were distributed according to the golden ratio. The band width of the seven colours – red, orange, yellow, green, blue, indigo, violet – are all different and follow each other to fit neatly into the band width of visible light. When you use the golden ratio to divide a line of a specific length, the seven sections will each occupy a different length of the line. From large to small, they occupy less and less space. The largest section occupies 39.55906% of the length of the entire line, the next 24.44888%, then 15.11025%, then 9.3386%, then 5.77156%, then 3.56707% and the smallest is 2.20455% long. In other words, it turns out that visible light is divided into seven colours, each of which take up a specific amount of space in the visible spectrum. The band width of the individual colours corresponds with the golden ratio as follows:

39.55906% – red

24.44888% – green

15.11025% – indigo

9.3386% – orange

---

[2] A colour is not one frequency. It is a range between a lower and an upper limit of frequency, which we call a bandwidth.

[3] A frequency is the number of times a complete wave repeats itself within a set time frame.

5.77156% – blue

3.56707% – violet

2.20455% – yellow

As you can see here:

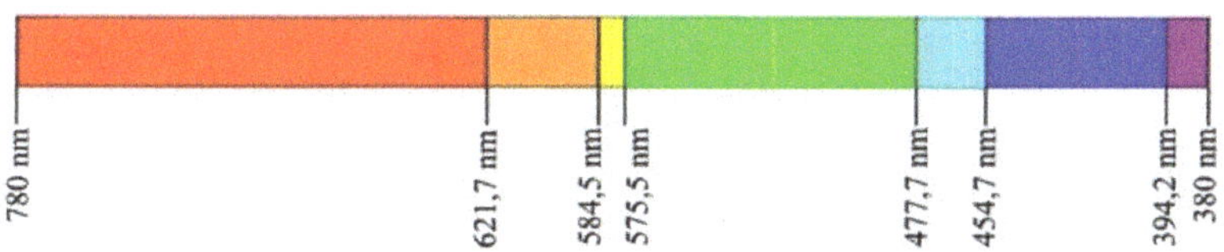

Let's quickly divert to the seven tissues of Ayurveda, I am particularly interested in these because I also know that in Eastern philosophy they talk about seven chakras[4] with each chakra being linked to one of the seven colours of the visible light spectrum. Perhaps there is a greater significance to all of this.

Ayurveda says that there are seven tissues, with each tissue originating out of the previous one, and that the process through which this happens is densification. The tissues, gradually, become more and more compact as we move from top to bottom. Let us put the list of seven tissues next to the list of seven colours:

Juices	red	39.6%
blood	green	24.4%
muscle	indigo	15.1%
fat	orange	9.3%
bone	blue	5.8%
nerve	violet	3.6%
seed	yellow	2.2%

---

[4] Chakras are the energy centres from which the physical structure of living organisms are constructed.

The first thing I noticed about this arrangement, taking the percentages into account, is that we are told the body is made up of two thirds water. Adding the first tissue (water), which makes up 39.6% of the total body, to the second one (thick water = blood), which makes up 24.4% of the total body, I get 64%. How much closer could you get to two thirds!

The other immediate conclusion from putting the two lists together has to be that the colours appear in a fixed order when visible light spreads out: first red, then green, then indigo, then orange, then blue, then violet and lastly yellow. This would appear to mean that everything could be constructed in seven layers, with the layers appearing in a predetermined way. Now we can take this scheme and go and measure everything in the universe, matching all aspects of creation using this basic formula. To my mind, the more we find that can be explained in these terms, the more we begin to believe there is some truth in it.

The code of life

From what you say, it seems that the number 7 is important in nature?

I'd say more than important. And then there is the Bible. The first thing the Bible talks about is creation. We are told creation happened in seven days. Right? Now I am interested! Again seven. However, in the Bible story creation as we know it stops at Day 6 and we are told that on the seventh day God rested. Isn't this strange?

Here is a way of understanding the story. On the first day heaven and earth were created. This refers to the separation of energies and matter. Heaven stands for the energies in the universe, the sky, and earth represents matter, the more solid parts of the universe. On day 2 the waters got separated from the land. Within matter, the more solid part of the universe, a division occurs between fluids and the actual solids such as rock. This completes the three states in which any matter can be observed, namely gas, liquid and solid. On day 3 plants arise. On day 4 simple egg-laying animals, large and small, appear. On day 5 mammals appear and on day 6 humans arrive. That is as far as creation has developed up to this point. In a sense, day 7 does exist but hasn't manifested yet. It is still to come, and we have no idea what that might entail.

The visible colours of light, the tissues of all living organisms and the Bible creation story can be aligned as follows:

red	juices/skin	heaven and earth
green	blood	water and land
indigo	muscle	plants
orange	fat	egg-laying animals
blue	bone	mammals
violet	nerve	humans
yellow	seed	?

As in life, as in creation, it is always the same construction, using the same seven layers. It would make sense to reference the layers by numbers rather than by descriptions. One way of doing that would be to look at the colours as they all have a fixed frequency band in a fixed specific order. The frequencies move from low to high passing the various colours in this particular order: from red to orange to yellow to green to blue to indigo to violet. If we attach a number to each of these then red becomes number 1, orange 2, yellow 3, green 4, blue 5, indigo 6 and violet 7.

From the colour sequence, as the visible light unfolds from one layer into the next, we have learned that the order in which the colours appear, also responsible for the amount of space they take up, is red – green – indigo – orange – blue – violet – yellow. The smallest of these energies, the last in the row, is a potential seed for creation. Our tests and calculations show that the creative seed only happens when yellow is last in the row. No other colour, energy frequency, has that power but it has to be in the right place. We deduce that our universe has been created out of a seed frequency from another existing universe. It broke open in the big bang and our universe started to unfold. It began to show the seven layers we have identified, in that specific order.

By numbering the colours, the numbers can be used to identify the sequence of events and the sequence of creation, whether it is the creation of colours, the universe or the tissues of organisms. Out of a seed from outside of the new creation a creation occurs from light to dense matter in seven stages, which can be represented by the following sequence 1-4-6-2-5-7-3. There you have the code of creation, the basic structure of all of our universe, expressed in a sequence of seven numbers, of which the last one, number 3, is the new seed for the creation of a new universe. The creation is like the Russian dolls called matryoshkas. Each manifestation is followed by the next, always structured in the same way. Interestingly, the matryoshka toy is made up of seven dolls.

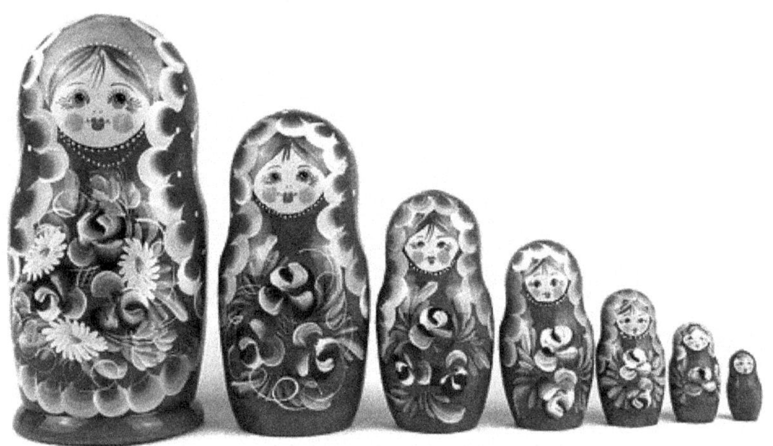

Every one of those seven layers is made up of something and has subdivisions. Since everything in the universe is created in seven layers and with these seven basic frequencies, the substructures also have to be a combination of these frequencies and layers.

Thank you for making it easy for my curious mind to comprehend. What is the composition of each colour? Are they also made up of seven layers?

-👆 We mustn't lose sight of the fact that our focus here is on health and what that means to individual people. Going into too much detail about the structure of the universe would be boring and beside the point. However, I am saying that the better you understand your world, and the universe, the more efficiently you can interact with it. I am going to make some statements about the structure and function of the universe based on our research as described in *Why Me? – Science and Spirituality as inevitable bed partners* (ISBN 978-90-827854-1-8).

What I have already shown you is that every part of creation has a seven-layered structure in which each subsequent layer emerges from the previous one and is more compact . This sequence is a direct result of the powers responsible for creation itself, lowering the temperature and increasing the pressure. Each of these subsequent layers has a smaller impact, occupies less space. Their contributions to the whole are expressed in the percentages I mentioned.

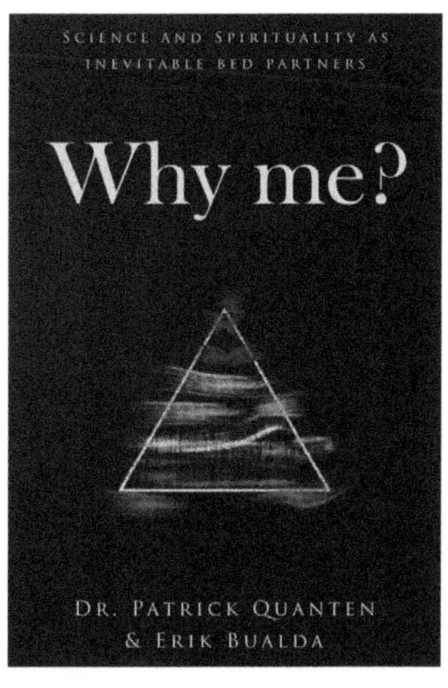

Everything in the universe must have the same basic structure and therefore we can use information we find within the microscopic world to explain something in the macroscopic world and vice versa. As it is inside so it will be outside. As it is above so it will be below. Here we can already conclude that whatever your world, your life, looks like on the outside it has a similar, comparable, structure and function on the inside. This is an important point with regards to health, but before going into all of that, there is another crucial question to answer.

Since everything in the universe is energy, everything in the universe is interconnected and everything in the universe is constantly in motion, how does energy exchange happen? Which energies play a major part and which play a minor part?

The problem in answering this question properly lies in the fact that energies cannot be pinned down to a place and time and therefore general conclusions cannot be drawn from observations made under very specific conditions. Using the principle that everything has the same structure and functions, according to the same principles, we found a way of solving this problem by investigating the "chakras" that are so important in Ayurvedic medicine.

The chakras

There are seven chakras, each one connected to a specific colour. These colours are represented in the same sequence of colours that are present in visible light, from 1 through to 7. Chakras are energy centres, nodules of energy that form gateways between the energetic form and the physical form. They function and connect as energy does, but these energy centres have very specific and fixed positions. Using the Golden Ratio, we were able to pinpoint each chakra in a specific place on the line connecting the base of the spine with the crown of the head. Measuring that distance allows us to accurately pinpoint the position of each chakra for each person. The chakras take up a relative position to one another that is the same for all human beings.

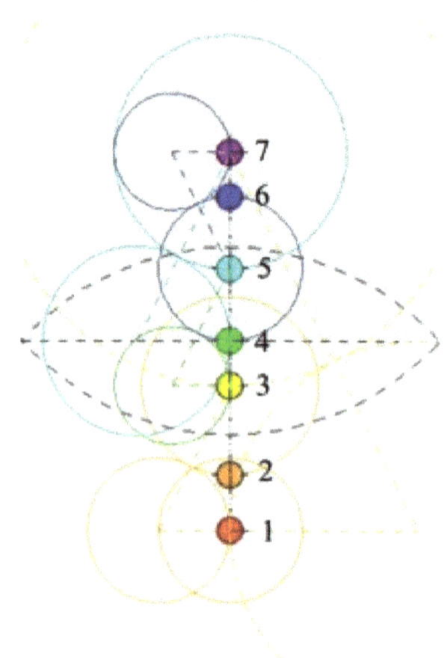

When we allow energy to flow from each of these chakras it

58

will spread into the universe and "hit" other chakras at set intervals, allowing them to exchange their information. Chakras that are closest to each other will receive more information and so influence each other much more than those further away. Using our knowledge about the beginning of creation, which is that from a seed energy, 3 energies 1 4 6 2 5 7 emerge before returning to 3, it can be seen that during the creative process the sequence of energy layers we encounter is 3-1-4-6-2-5-7-3. These can be placed in that order on the chakra positions as this is the order in which they have appeared during the creative process.

From this we can determine the impact of each chakra on all the other chakras during creation. We can determine what its impact is on the structure and function of the other chakras. The impact will show us the contribution each chakra, and therefore each energy layer, has on the other ones. Let's jump to the result of these observations.

In this figure we can see that by drawing concentric circles for each chakra centred on chakra 1, we first meet 1 than 3 than 4 then 6 then 2 then 5 and lastly 7. For chakra 4, the next in the creation sequence, the influence is distributed throughout the chakras 4-6-1-2-3-5-7, as demonstrated by the concentric circles in the following illustration.

When we look at 6, the next step in evolution, we find that there are two possibilities: 6-4-2-1-5 and then it can be either 3-7 or 7-3 (as illustrated). The information leaving chakra 6 reaches chakras 3 and 7 at the same time. Hence, either one can be dominant over the other.

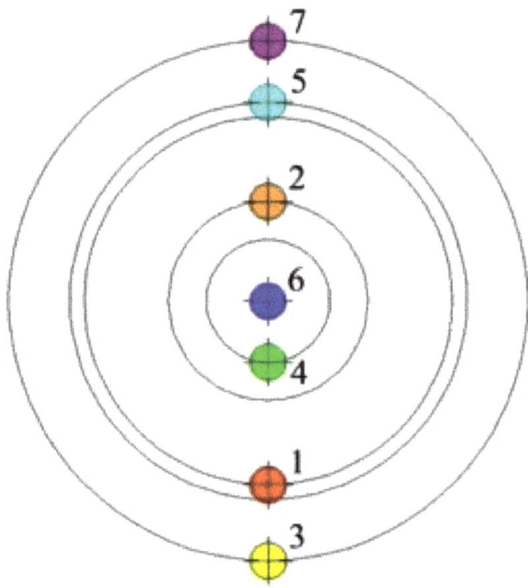

It turns out that the frequency split in 6 is creating a bottom half (3-7) and a top half (7-3). That manifests firstly in the chakras themselves and then later on also in physical manifestations. So, the chakras, and everything that follows on, now have an upper and a bottom part. At this point in evolution, physical manifestation also gets a different top part from the bottom part.

For 2, it is even more complicated because outgoing from chakra 2 the information reaches, in the first instance, chakras 5 and 6 at the same time, which creates two possible lines of ordering the information. At the next level, we can see that the information reaches chakras 4 and 7 at the same time, once again causing a further split, creating even more options for the physical manifestations.

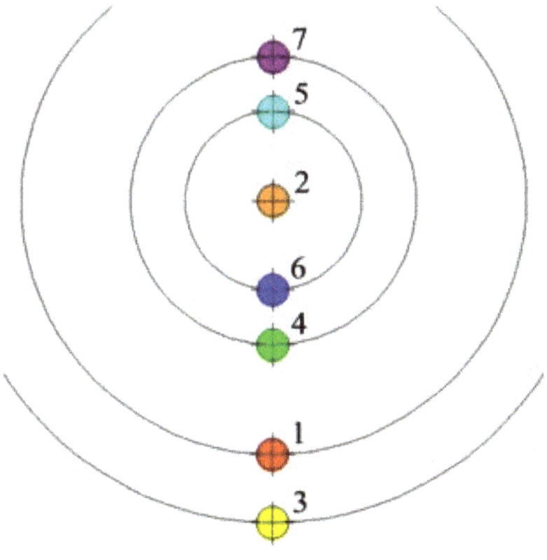

2-6-5-4-7-1-3   2-5-6-4-7-1-3

2-6-5-7-4-1-3   2-5-6-7-4-1-3

By centring the concentric circles on the remaining chakras, 3, 5 and 7, we have the following sequences:

3-1-4-6-2-5-7

5-7-2-6-4-1-3

7-5-2-6-4-1-3

The different ways of possibly combining frequencies in order to end up with the same frequency band in, for instance, frequency 2, must show up somewhere in physical manifestation too. The different combinations are noticeable as divisions within the chakras themselves and from there on also in the physical manifestations that follow the flow of energy through the chakras. A split within a chakra manifests as two "different" physical manifestations. These are the same in tissues but different in layout. For instance, the split which occurs in chakra 6 (the combination is either 3-7 or 7-3) leads to a differentiation within the physical form of the living organism, which now manifests a different top half and bottom half. The first level split in 2 manifests as a different front and back of the organism, while the next split level in 2 manifests as a different left and right side to the organism. After completion of these splits the chakras are receiving information from the outside world through eight different "filters': top left front and right front, top left back and right back, and the same four in the bottom part of the chakras. These filters are making slight nuances to the energy flowing through the chakras, in the sense that one part of the chakra will emphasize 6 more than 5, and so on. This also modifies physical manifestation of living organisms as a result of what is happening in the chakras.

The creation of the universe can now be considered in more detail:

Day 1	Frequency 1	Heaven and earth
Day 2	Frequency 4	Water and land
Day 3	Frequency 6	Plants – bottom (roots) differs from top (plant)
Day 4	Frequency 2	Egg laying animals – first difference between left and right and then between back and front, where we see in some animals the development of a spine, a skeleton (5 before 6)
Day 5	Frequency 5	Mammals – differences between the front and back parts of the body but with some correspondence between them
Day 6	Frequency 7	Humans – differences between the top and bottom halves of the body but with some correspondence between them
Day 7	Frequency 3	?

We now also know that frequency 1 is a combination of 1-3-4-6-2-5-7, with frequency 1 contributing 39,55906% down to frequency

7 contributing 2,20455%. And every frequency can be divided into their seven coloured layers.

In terms of physical matter, we can classify the matter created per biblical day as follows:

Day 1 *atoms – seven layers*

- halogens and noble gas
- non-metals
- alkali and alkaline earth metals
- metalloids
- transition metals
- lanthanide
- actinide

Day 2 *molecules – seven layers*

- covalent molecules
- ionic molecules
- carbohydrates
- lipids
- amino acids
- proteins
- nucleic acids

And so on…

The reason there are different colours and that the colours are related to individual chakras is because they each represent something different. Each chakra has a different "meaning", a different content. Many books have been written about the meanings of different chakras, and what they stand for, but I will try and keep it simple so we can develop our thinking and understanding. In a simple way, the meaning of each colour and frequency can be defined as follows:

1. form

2. movement

3. personal power

4. balance

5. communication

6. consciousness

7. knowledge

These basic layers of the energetic field can each be seen to bring information of a specific kind to life. This can be traced to the non-material part of life as well as the material part. These are the seven parts of life, the way each organism has been created. They are also the seven types of information that run through physical creation, those which make it function. Each organism, and specimen of each organism has been created in a very specific way so that within each colour and information layer, the organism has balance. Once this organism with its specific balance gets exposed to the influx of information from the surrounding world then that influx becomes its feeding ground. This influx either strengthens the organism or weaken it. This forms the basis of health and illness.

Balance is the key

This has all been very theoretical and not easy to assimilate. Does this knowledge about chakras affect our health? To put it in another way, do we need to know all this in order to be healthy?

⬧ Let's go with the theory for a little longer and then I can give you better answers. The point here is that all matter has been built in seven layers with seven different frequencies of information, each layer made up out of the same seven frequencies only in different proportions. For example, when we compare the makeup of frequency 1, we have 1-3-4-6-2-5-7, and for frequency 7, we have 7-5-2-6-4-1-3. In frequency 1 frequency 7 only represents 2,2% while in frequency 7 it represents 39,6%. This placing in the order of the code tells us how much of that specific information is present within the manifestation, according to the golden ratio.

Let's have a look at what else evolution shows us. On day 3, frequency 6, we know that there are two ways of composing 6. The sequence ending on 7 manifests as the solid parts of creation within this universe. In these seven layers the first one is a lot lighter than the rest of the layers and then they get progressively more dense, as follows:

- magma
- minerals, crystals
- igneous rock
- sedimentary rock
- metamorphic rock
- cumulate rock
- source rock

The sequence ending on 3, however, produces a new structure called a cell. The first, and most primitive, cell that manifests in this form is called a prokaryote. This will evolve, become more complex and refined in its structures, becoming a form called a eukaryote. From this a plant cell evolves, and later an animal cell. That gives rise to the manifestation of egg laying animals, to invertebrates and vertebrates. Later in evolution the eukaryote develops into a mammal cell and later still into a human cell. The organisms that grow out of such cells, in turn develop seven functional systems, which we can also mark as 1-4-6-2-5-7-3 (the code of creation). Science has now proven that these systems already exist within the singular cell from which they develop. Every cell has, in miniature, the same seven systems every living organism develops, and they are:

1. lymphatic system
2. circulation system
3. feeding system (breathing and digestion)

4. mobility system
5. sensory system
6. nervous system
7. glandular system

Each of these are, in turn, made up of the same seven frequencies, the same atoms and molecules, as the original cell. For instance, we can look at frequency 2, the mobility system and recognise seven subdivisions in the structure of the skeleton, each of which is made up out of the same seven layers.

1. tail
2. pelvis, hips, legs
3. lower back
4. chest, ribs
5. shoulders, arms
6. neck, face
7. skull

That means that when there is a problem with the balance of one of these frequencies, as is the case in illness, then that will have its effect in ALL systems, in other words, all through the body and mind of the organism. This may show up as outside, visible or noticeable, signs in different organs but they are all part of the same imbalance. This is an homeopathic principle!

Do you mean that all the symptoms and all the characteristics of a person are connected and have only one source in them?

➨ This is the practical aspect that you asked me about in your last question. Homeopathy is not looking for a cure for a person's headache. It is looking to restore their balance. Consequently, the remedy used for one person's headache may be totally different from the remedy for another person's headache.

If we want to actively intervene in the balance of our health and disease it would be wise to understand that everything in the universe is connected and that every part of the body and mind is made of the same energies, frequencies and information. This means that a specific rock or fluid or gas can contain a high percentage of a certain specific energy that the system and/or the molecules within the human body will respond to, wherever that energy is highest or most prominent.

Solid matter such as rock radiates energy on a more permanent and long term basis while fluids are more easily changed and gasses only deliver energy fleetingly. It is this principle that homeopathy uses in delivering its message of a remedy in water. Precious stones and precious metals, gold and silver, have been used for many thousands of years to help stabilize and balance individual lives. This also explains why people from certain regions on earth have similar characteristics. They all grew up exposed to the same radiation.

Put more generally, our environment feeds us with information, energies, that will resonate within the tissues of the body and the frequencies of the mind. At any given time, those frequencies have a balance point. In the universe that point changes with evolution and so the information input from one era is not the same as the input from another. Each individual, however, has a balance point that has become fixed once the basic maturation process has come to an end.

The cell has information in every colour, but it is much more specific than that. The information within every colour is limited too. The entire frequency band is not manifested within the physical, within the cell, only a very specific small range of that frequency. Then the surrounding feeding grounds, firstly the mother during pregnancy and later family and the human world, modify this to a specific balance point. Further input from an ever-changing world and universe will put a strain on this balance point which might show itself as diseases. Since these same frequencies are present in all parts of our mental and physical makeup, imbalances can show up in many places, but we will have to remember that there really is only one imbalance.

Find the imbalance and it will be simple to cure the manifested diseases by rectifying the imbalance. In practice it turns out that it may be simple – but it certainly won't be easy! The reason for this is that it frequently requires us to make fundamental changes to the way we have been leading our lives up to that point, the point where illness showed itself.

From what you are saying, it is increasingly clear to me how lost we human beings are in this time, searching for health in material things, in external medicines, and putting our lives in the hands of people who do not deserve our trust. There are many devious people on earth right now, too many. Might it be that the energies that are coming in from the vibrations we are receiving from the universe are distorted? Might we be being affected by some evil energy field? Or is this putting the cause back in the outside world?

Indeed. In creation there are no evil forces. Everything has a purpose, a life with a beginning and an end. Creation is a constant transformation. All influences are needed in order for momentum to continue. The judgement of good and bad is a human illusion that no other creature shares with us. It is part of that frequency 7 that we are being created from. Do not forget that humanity is still in its infancy and has developed little since the development of mammals.

Disease occurs when there is an ongoing discrepancy between inner constitutional and learned patterns, and outer environmental patterns. This discrepancy leads to change. Either you become ill and die or you change. Disease is a natural phenomenon that is our guide in life, something we can embrace and shouldn't be fighting. If we were able to work with disease we would learn more quickly and be happier. It is fear, fear of an enemy and a danger that is not present not real and that creates unhappiness.

Creation as it has happened until now, and we cannot know anything more, has happened in 6 "days". The Fibonacci series show the figures 0, 1, 1, 2, 3, 5, 8, 13, ... (Golden Ratio). From zero and one another one is created. This one force, the unity, creates two forces in the universe. The first force is fire, the creative "element". This creates two opposing forces, expansion and contraction. Together they form the Holy Trinity. And as mentioned before the three forces then create five elements, which in turn create seven tissues, plus an eighth one which is the same as the first one but in seed form. These are the physical manifestations. That is when everything on all levels has been completed, which at this point in time it has not.

In Western music there are seven full notes that are combined in an octave, a complete set of seven plus the next note, which is a repeat from the first one, put one step lower. There are seven colours to the visible spectrum as there are seven musical notes. However, their combination is in a set of eight. On top of that, there are five semitones within the same octave. They are separate notes but aren't quite full. Yet, although they are not full, they certainly belong to the octave, which brings the total number of steps from the beginning of one octave to the end of that octave to thirteen. These semitones are organised in a set of two and a set of three.

There are also five parts of the visible light spectrum that are not visible, not a fully manifested part, but together they make up the entire spectrum. Two infrared bands and three ultraviolet bands belong to the visible spectrum.

While creation is a work in progress, we can see what the completed structure will look like, even if we do not know the details of what will manifest. We know what frequencies belong where and what kinds of information they hold.

One of the seven bodily tissues you mentioned is seed. I have been looking for this expression in medical books but have not found it anywhere. It seems that Western medicine considers four fundamental types of tissues: epithelial, connective, muscular and nervous, plus a few secondary tissues. In effect, I have not found a consensus on the exact number of tissues we have in the human body. Those I have found are epithelial lining, connective, nervous, smooth muscle, striated muscle, cardiac muscle, epithelial, glandular, sensory epithelial, adipose, bone, blood, haematopoietic,

cartilaginous and lymphatic tissues. None of them fit into what you are calling seed tissue. It is a rather strange concept in my language, Spanish. Would you clarify what you mean?

 Of course. It is not only strange in Spanish! In English it is also strange to use the word seed in this context. However, the meaning of this word is exactly what we mean and that is why I use it. As we have seen in this chapter, every possible combination of the seven frequencies contains the frequency 3. Frequency 3 means "inner power" and when it is presented in its most compact form, placed in the last position in the row of frequencies, the higher pressure results in the appearance of a new specimen, perhaps a new oak tree, a new human being or a new breed. It depends on the level at which that "seed" sprouts. These are the pillars on which everything new within creation begins, hence the name seed.

What does Western medicine call this type of tissue? Or haven't they realised it exists?

 That must be it. They just haven't noticed. As far as we know, no one else is studying the seven energetic layers that make up the structure of the universe. The word tissue is not a physical manifestation, as believed by the medical profession, but, as we use it, it indicates the potential of that frequency band at that particular level of universal development. In other words, it is only when the development of the universe has reached the level for living creatures to be formed that we use the word tissue in a physical sense.

The names of the seven tissues I mentioned earlier, therefore, do not refer to the physical presence of animal tissues. They refer to the potential of these seven different energies and their characteristics. At the next level of development, the same seven frequencies are called "systems", and are given the names that best reflect the characteristic potentials of these frequencies.

In some traditions it is common practice name an energetic phenomenon with a word derived from something physical that exemplifies the characteristics of that energy. In both Ayurveda and Chinese medicine, the names given to the elements (ether, air, fire, water, earth) are not derived from their physical presence, but rather are indicative of the main characteristics on which the elements – energetics – are based. In the same way, the images of Heaven or the Garden of Eden are concepts that do not have a physical manifestation either, just as the Tree of Life does not have a physical manifestation.

Philosophy is free
and the physician must be a philosopher,
not a sectarian.

Knowledge does not consist
in following in the footsteps of the Master,
but in knowing things by their causes
and distinguishing the black from the white.

Sheep are to be pitied,
if one goes after the other,
because the shepherds lead them by force,
and they lack the use of reason.

But that men, absolute in genius
and free in their knowledge,
run after the dictates of others
is a deplorable weakness of human understanding.

Yesterday and Today.
El mundo engañado por los falsos medicos
Extract from the book

III

THE ORIGIN OF DISEASES

We have put on the table that disease is an imbalance between the two aspects of our system: matter and energy. When you talk about imbalance, I imagine a pair of scales that can tip to the right or to the left depending on the weight you put on it. Is disease, or imbalance, also like this? Can it go to one side or the other?

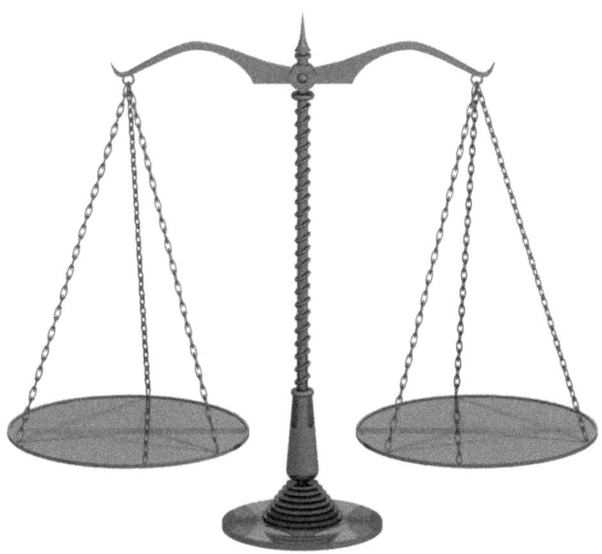

➤ Health is balance and disease is imbalance, but the image of a pair of scales does not work. Firstly, the scale is a fixed entity and although we can agree on scales being differently and individually made, they are always the same. They never change, and that is not the case with the balance of health in life. Secondly, with a scale you can put weights on one side and it will have a direct effect on the other side, but this is not the same in life. We require a different image for the ever-changing system of balance in life.

Every part of creation has properties we can measure and observe because it is made that way. The properties of a particular life are present and detectable within the structure of that life. The property of being protected against too much heating from the sun is reflected in some people's dark skin. The property of being able to jump high is reflected in long legs and a high pelvis. Once we have a fixed structure like a physical body, the properties and characteristics are fixed into a limited band of possible changes. If one pushes the structure any further it will break or disintegrate. The kind of image we need is one with a limited but real flexibility band. Balance is a range of frequencies, of possibilities, within the limits of the structure of the living organism.

You can compare this to non-living matter in the sense that the construction of water as a liquid has its limitations. When it gets too warm the liquid evaporates and disappears into gas. When it gets too cold the liquid disappears into ice, the solid form of water. Either way water no longer flows and no longer exists in its liquid form.

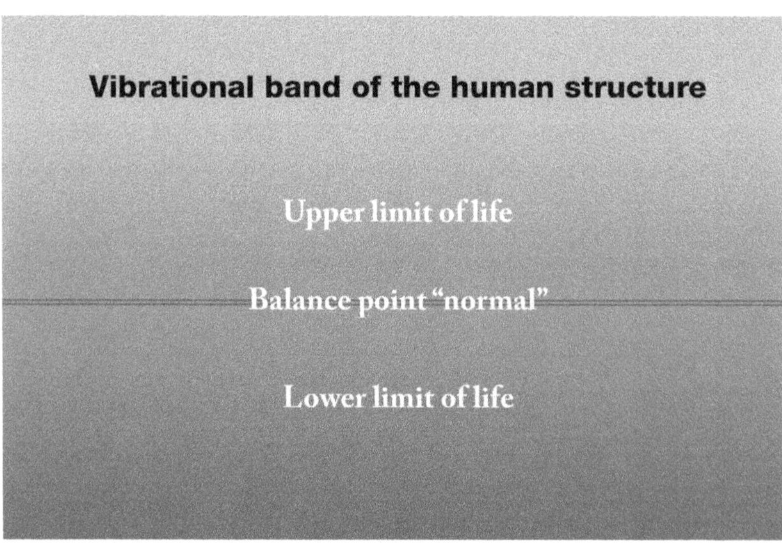

The human physical construction, which comes from an energetic field, also has an upper and a lower limit. Within this limit life as we know it is possible. In the middle of this limit lies the balance point, which in fact is a small band of what we might call normal for that individual. Between the edge of the normal band and the end of life band lies a grey area in which life within the structure is still possible but not as smooth as within the balance band.

Compare it with the water structure. There is a small density band of water in which water is in balance whereby the forces that keep that balance are the least strained. Water flows easily, without effort. A change in temperature will not immediately lead to the disappearance of the liquid water form. First the density will adjust a little. This will make flow a little more difficult but still possible. A bigger change in temperature will result in the disintegration of the liquid physical structure.

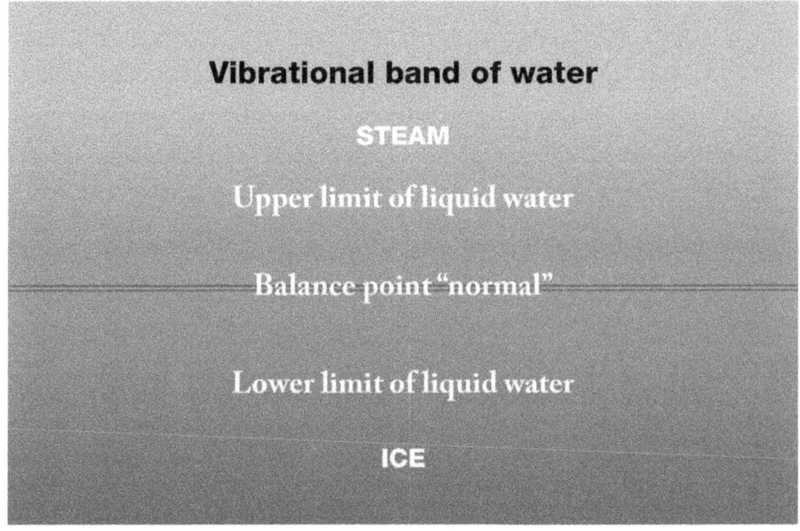

To visualise balance in life we need a density scale. In the illustration below we can shift the frequency from point C to C' and still maintain the same structure, but beyond that the structure as we know it, the physical form of a human being, will disintegrate.

The scales are individually built, they have a flexible balance band at the centre and they have end limitations in both directions.

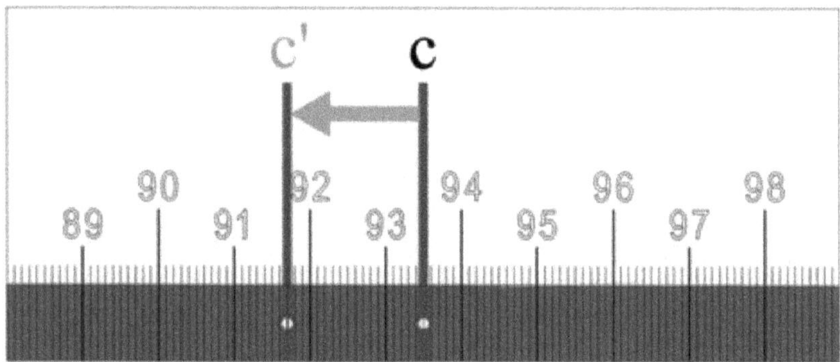

The other difference between this image and the traditional scales is the fact that we are not putting weights on one side or the other. When we are talking about a density scale, the shift that occurs is a shift within the same spectrum towards a higher density or towards a lower density. Hence it is only a shift in how compact the structure is within the band that allows it to live. Beyond that, life as we know it ceases.

The only things that can influence the structure and the balance of the life within that structure are things that have constructed this life and fixed the energies into a specific form. That form has been a result of two forces that worked on the original energetic field.

Temperature and pressure

Only a change in temperature and/or a change in pressure will cause the balance of a life to shift. Hence, anything that has an influence on the temperature and/or pressure of a living structure has an influence on the balance of that structure.

Health is a balance in life. That balance is *an individual issue.* That balance is changed by everything in creation as it has been made in the same way out of the same basic existing energy. Everything will exert influence through a change in temperature and/ or pressure. An imbalance can be caused in any one of the seven subdivisions of life, and that will distort and disturb life, the fixed structure.

Do you mean to say that when we get sick it's because our temperature or pressure has changed? Is it that simple?

◗ Everything is created because of a reduction in temperature and an increase in pressure. Energy condenses so much that it becomes manifest, which means that all of creation is a specific state of density, the state we can observe. The rest of non-material creation, the energetic fields, functions in exactly the same way, but outside of our physical observation range. We don't get any information on it because our senses cannot directly connect with those densities. Material creation is about the density of energies. This means that our bodies are also a condensation of energies, densities of a very particular range. Each person occupies a specific place on the entire density spectrum of what manifests as human beings. Everything in creation is constructed in seven layers. And it is the harmony in each of those layers and the harmony between them that keeps it together, maintains the shape, and allows energy to flow through, without the flow bursting its banks. Changing the density of this harmonious structure will make it malfunction and eventually dissociation will occur. Think about the harmony that keeps a champagne glass in its shape and form and how that can suddenly burst and shatter into thousands of pieces simply under the influence of Ella Fitzgerald's singing voice. The influence of that energetic wave disturbed the balance, the resonant frequency, within the glass structure to the extent that it was no longer able to keep its structure.

There are seven different types of information, seven different energy bands, each with specific information:

1.	form
2.	mobility
3.	personal power
4.	balance
5.	communication
6.	consciousness
7.	knowledge

These correspond to the seven functional systems:

1.	form	lymphatic and skin
2.	mobility	motility
3.	personal power	glandular
4.	balance	circulatory
5.	communication	sensory
6.	consciousness	nutritional (breathing and digestion)
7.	knowledge	nervous

Each of these systems is made up of the same seven tissues:

1.	form	lymphatic and skin	juices/water
2.	mobility	motility	fat
3.	personal power	glandular	seed
4.	balance	circulatory	blood
5.	communication	sensory	bone
6.	consciousness	nutritional	muscle
7.	knowledge	nervous	nerve

These tissues are made up from these atomic and molecular structures:

1	form	lymphatic and skin	juices/water	atoms
2	mobility	motility	fat	lipids
3	personal power	glandular	seed	nucleic acids
4	balance	circulatory	blood	simple molecules
5	communication	sensory	bone	amino acids
6	consciousness	nutritional	muscle	carbohydrates
7	knowledge	nervous	nerve	proteins

There is a harmony between all manifestations on all levels of the human body, which means that there is only a small range of frequencies for each of the seven layers in which the complex structure can maintain its balance and function easily. When a frequency gets pushed beyond its harmony limits it puts a strain on the entire structure. A "change in frequency" is not really a change in frequency. It is actually a change in density that the frequency is experiencing. The more dense and compact the frequency becomes the slower it will travel. This manifests in harder tissues, in more compact tissues and in heavier tissues. This in turn means that the function of those tissues has now become slower and less effective than before. Then it requires much more effort, more energy, to complete normal tasks. The tissues are becoming diseased and eventually all life will stop flowing through them.

Disease or disharmony happens because of the influence of temperature and pressure on the energies. Notice that when frequency 4 gets disrupted and changes its density it changes the complexion of simple molecules like the water molecule or salt molecules. It might also the manifestation of the blood tissue. This could show itself as circulatory problems within that specific human being. On an energetic level this person probably has difficulty maintaining a balance between his own needs and the demands of others. This is, in a nut-shell, how it happens. Why is a different matter.

What you are saying is that when a frequency is disturbed and pushed beyond its harmonic limits, it puts a strain on the entire structure and that is when illness appears. What is it that disturbs the frequencies to such an extent? What is the source of this distortion and at what level does it occur?

➥ The construction of one human specimen occurs over a very short time and happens in three stages that cover three layers. All three layers are to be fixed within the limits of the particular life that is to be formed.

- The deepest and first layer is built with information from genetic material.

- The second layer gets its information from the mother. The foetus builds tissues in a harmonic structure that prepares it for the world the way the mother experiences it.

- The third layer is built with information the child receives from its direct interactions with the new world it enters. This layer is more or less a "functional outside", an expression of the structure of the deeper layers.

In essence, the body is no more than frequencies fixed in a series of narrow bands. There are two characteristics to every frequency band at every level in all places.

One is the width of the band. The narrower the band is the more "fixed" the structure is, meaning that there is not much room for flexibility, for much "give and take". This information, this frequency, becomes strained very quickly when there is even a slight a slight deviation from balance. The second characteristic is the intensity of the frequency, the amplitude. You can visualise this as the hue of a colour. It may be very bright and harsh or be a pastel shade.

To make it easier to understand, we can use the example of sound. The loudness of the sound is the intensity, the amplitude of the sound. How high or low the note is, is the frequency of the sound. Of course, every human being is built with specific information that belongs to a very specific time, to a very specific place and very specific circumstances. The frequencies a child has fixed in its tissues are constantly moving. *Nothing stays the same in life.* Life is a constant interaction between the inner world of a person (the fixed structure) their outer world, the human world, the natural world and the universe. The changes in the outer world are of two kinds:

- intensities (amplitudes) of each of the frequencies
- the balance between the contributions of each frequency to the whole, the band width.

Changes in amplitude are easy to spot because they can be seen in the material world as a change in temperature, in humidity, in numbers. These are basically changes in the intensity of whatever is already there.

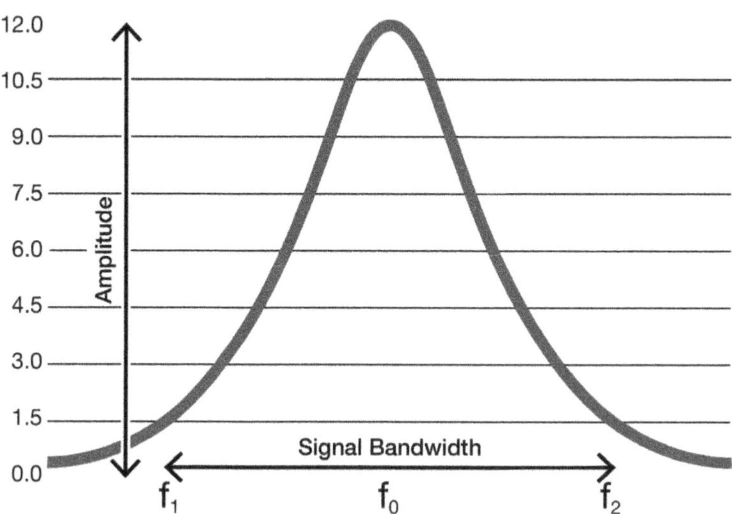

Changes in the contribution to the balance of each of the seven frequencies means that there is a change in emphasis. During one era of human history the emphasis is on travel and during another on communication. These are changes in the balance of the universe, resulting in different phases of universal development. This example demonstrates a shift from frequency 2 towards frequency 5:

2	mobility	movement system	fat tissue	fats
5	communication	sensory system	bone tissue	amino-acids

These changes are cyclical and progressive, following a pattern of creation which flows out of the unfolding of the frequencies as laid out in the creation code. The entire universe, and everything in it, manifested and unmanifested, is an expression of the same seven frequencies.

As human beings, part of the fixed manifested matter in the universe, we are surrounded by the various layers out of which we have sprung. We can identify some of them easily as family, community, village or city, race, humanity, animals, plants, earth, solar system, milky way, cosmos. Each layer has its own time frame and its own cycles. Hence, at any given moment in time at each of those universal levels there is a preponderance of expression of a specific frequency, and those layers are at different stages of development. The layers closest to the individual have the greatest impact on their life but all do have an impact.

What kind of impact?

Each of the seven inner frequencies responds and communicates with the same frequencies on the outside. That happens on all the levels of our construction. It is how the manifested part gets fed, how the flow of life through the manifested part is sustained.

Expansion and contraction

When the intensity of the communication frequency in our surroundings increases, an expression of frequency 5, that pressure will be felt everywhere in our system. In human constructions, where communication is a weak part of the structure, it may cause malfunctioning. This can cause physical manifestations in the neck and shoulders, (frequency 5 within the mobility system), in breathing and digestion, in the skin, and so on.

When the outside world evaluates certain frequencies as more important, a change in band width, even greater problems emerge in the manifested fixed world. For example, when the balance shifts towards a greater emphasis on frequency 1 in the earth manifestation we are subjected to more flooding, resulting in many more people's structures becoming defunct, which can cause more people to die. Particular people will be unable to make room for this expansion of frequency 1 because of the limited "space "they have in their structures and their systems will cease to function. This is an exchange of information between the outer world and the inner world. There is an interaction. It is not simply the existence of a certain situation or condition that is "good" or "bad", but it is a certain situation that will *favour* specific constructions, in this case human beings with specific characteristics, who have enough bandwidth of that particular frequency at their disposal to absorb the shift.

A change in intensity will lead to either a contraction, an increased density of the tissue, which will make the flow of energy through the tissues, in other words living, more difficult, or to an expansion. There is a lower limit, below which too little energy can get through and life ceases. There is also an upper limit to the expansion which will allow the energy to flow much more easily. This results in too expansive a field so that the structure loses its shape. Then life within that environment is no longer possible because the flow of energy is not sufficiently directed. When energy flow disperses, life disperses.

An alteration of the frequency bandwidth results in a change in the type of tissue. When a fixed structure can no longer contain a frequency within the limits of the bandwidth it has available for that frequency it can only carry on by switching to the next frequency.

This may be difficult to imagine. Let me give you a practical example. You change one aspect of your interaction with the outside world: you start to drink a lot of whiskey. Soft tissue cells of the liver belong in the category of frequency 6 (muscle tissue in Ayurveda). By drinking a lot of alcohol you change the environment of these cells and eventually you will see a change happening within your liver cells. They become fatty (frequency 2 – fat tissue) instead of frequency 6, as they originally were. Your doctor will do tests and warn you your liver is turning fatty. But you continue creating the same environment for your liver cells and, after some time, your doctor will tell you that you have liver cirrhosis, which is a hardening of the liver cells (frequency 5 – bone tissue). Now remember the creation code 1-4-6-2-5-7-3. Under the pressure of the outside changed environment – you weren't built for this – your tissues try to survive by shifting frequencies in order to "absorb" that pressure. They go from soft (6), to less soft (2), to hard (5).

A living system will try and absorb changes at all levels, whenever it can shift a bit within a frequency. This means that ongoing stress will show itself in one person in a certain part of their body and bodily function, while for someone else the initial sign will be in a different part or function .For example, sadness can cause one person headaches, another digestive problems and a third one heartache.

As the circumstances remain or worsen, signs will occur in other places and in other functions as a direct result of the same frequency changes being expressed in different body parts. This is also why we can see infections "spreading" to specific places, for example from bladder to kidney or from throat to lungs. This is why we see tumours (metastases – secondaries) appear in parts of the body that are distant from the first one. This is why eczema and asthma are so often seen together in children. They are different expressions of the same frequencies in different parts or functions of the body.

The origin of the changes within the structure of a human being, lies in the interaction between the individual and the environment.

The mere presence of a situation or condition is not enough for anything to happen to them. It requires reactions to the outside environment that will allow changes to take place. Then another important aspect of this interaction comes into play. That is that for the inner world to formulate a response our cells are equipped with "antennae" in order to pick up information from the outside world. As the cell, and the entire organism, needs to survive in the outside world it requires all potentially life-threatening information to pass through. However, the human being also has frequency receivers, antennae, that can be switched on or off. In other words, we have the capacity to decide what information we will listen to and what not. We do not have to listen to everything. This is like deciding you do not want to hear the news, so you don't switch on the television or radio. We have a capacity to do the same in life. Information that does not enter the cells does not have to be dealt with, does not require a response, does not have an influence on the balance of our inner frequencies.

The "fixed" frequencies within the physical structure have limitations as to the variation in amplitude as well as the frequency bandwidth. There is only so much noise we can literally stand. There is only so much sharpness, so much movement, so much knowledge each of us individually can cope with. That refers to the amplitude range. Just as a crystal glass can shatter when exposed to a certain sound, so too can the physical tissues of the body "break" when their energetic tolerance limits are exceeded. The limits of the amplitude, intensity, of incoming signals are set by the tolerance of the tissues, fixed energies, of the individual to these signals. Each person is limited with respect to what their system can withstand, in all aspects of life, before the system, body and mind, begins to malfunction. Physically, these limitations manifest themselves, for example, in the range of motion, muscle strength, sensory sensitivity, digestive power and respiratory capacity. For example, we can't stand a noise that is too loud or a light that is too bright. Our range of movement is limited, and so is the amount of knowledge we can handle. Each individual has his or her own limitations.

On the other hand, the bandwidth allows for some slight changes to frequencies. Each frequency shifts within its own bandwidth. Close to the edges of that bandwidth the "clarity" of the signal begins to fade, but we still receive the message and we still recognise it as being that frequency. Our system will be able to identify which is the main frequency of that information, the main content of the message, and therefore will be able to respond to the stimulus in an appropriate way. If the variations in these frequencies exceed certain limits, signals will no longer be understandable to our systems, and therefore will not be able to respond appropriately. This is like the frequency scale on an old radio transistor. At a certain frequency you received the radio signal loud and clear. Alter the frequency slightly to the left or to the right and you will start to get interference, muddling the signal. Go even further and the signal begins to break up. So, staying "in tune" with one's environment is vital in order to be able to communicate clearly with the outside world. Long periods of alterations in those two parameters will change the functions of cells and therefore of the organism.

No doubt you are aware that these approaches are, to put it mildly, novel as well as initially difficult to assimilate. Let me ask you to summarise please. Are all manifested things related to the seven basic energies and is our health is based on the interplay of these energies?

➤ Don't worry, I'll try to explain it differently. Yes, in the manifested world there are just seven different energies. First, the universe manifests holding these energies. The most dense, most contracted, most compressed parts, will become "matter". Matter gradually manifests because of increased pressure on the energies. More and more compacted matter appears from atoms to small molecules to more complex molecules like proteins. There are seven layers of basic building blocks.

When we get to the third layer where solids are becoming manifest there occurs a split as part of the solids form cells, different structures from simply compacted solids. The split happens here because in frequency 6, the third layer, there are two equal possibilities for energy to be expressed (6-4-2-1-5-3-7 or 6-4-2-1-5-7-3). The line of simple solids evolves further within the universe to complete seven layers, but a side line development is now starting.

A very primitive cell, first layer, develops into more complex and active unicellular organisms like bacteria, second layer, and later into primitive plant cells, third layer. At this level a split occurs because once again we have reached frequency 6. On one line plants develop to fill the seven layers of the cell universe and on the side line animal cells arrive.

From primitive animal cells all egg-laying animals develop, again in seven layers. The first animals to develop are invertebrates up to the third level, where again a split occurs. This development in the animal sphere evolves further to complete the seven layers, from this point on with vertebrates, egg-laying animals. The side line sees the beginning of mammals.

From primitive mammals different layers develop, as with every layer that has gone before, according to the manifestation code 1-4-6-2-5-7-3.

Human beings begin their development at frequency 6 in the mammal universe.

There are three states of manifestation, gas, liquid and solid – and there are splits within the developing universe – cells in plants, animals, mammals, humans. All manifestations are combinations of seven different energies.

The human being is a split part of the mammal sphere, which is "surrounded" by the egg-laying animal sphere, which is surrounded by the cell sphere, which is surrounded by the universe, just like Russian dolls. Mammals and human beings are dependent upon the feeding, the support, of the sphere they are a part of, which is to a large extent insects. Their universe is part of and depends on the support of the bacterial universe. The outermost layer is the universe with its cosmic influences.

The closer the layer of a universe is the greater its impact on the creation of the sphere that holds and supports it. This means that the earth is influenced directly by energies from outer space.

Humanity is directly influenced by energies from the animal world and changes that happen on that level. In essence, the changes that happen at any level are alterations in one or more of those seven different energies. When, for instance, energy 5 changes, contracts and becomes more compact, then that will have a contracting and compacting energy 5 effect wherever that energy has manifested in creation. It won't affect everywhere in the same way because it depends how important energy 5 is in a specific construction. Energy 5 is the first of the seven energies in the code for the mammal universe and so any change in 5 will have a massive effect there, while energy 1 is only present in a small portion (5-7-2-6-4-1-3) in that specific manifestation.

It is important to remember that everything is made of the same seven frequencies, energies, but in different proportions and combinations. Any change at whatever level of a particular frequency will have an effect throughout the entire universe, in all layers.

Every frequency itself is a band of energy with, on one side, the more compact part, and on the other side the less compact part. Each manifestation in the material universe only shows a very limited part of that frequency and has a specific place within the width of the frequency band. For example, some people are built with a frail body and others with a robust one. Some people have heavy bones and thick muscles while others have lighter bones and thinner muscles, but these are all manifestations of muscles and bones, with the same frequencies.

A specific physical manifestation is a fixed portion of the energy bandwidth of that frequency, that energy. Because it is only a small fraction of the entire scope of that energy, it must be obvious that when the main pressure in that energy field begins to shift away from the part that is manifested and fixed within the organism that such a shift would put a lot of pressure on the organism. We call the manifestation of this pressure shift disease. It is an imbalance between the small range of flexibility and adaptability the physical organism has compared with the far greater flexibility of the entire field. When a frequency in our environment changes, our system, or more precisely that part of our system that is the manifestation of that specific energy, becomes seriously pressurised, ill and out of balance.

The universe is in motion and evolving all the time. This results in balance changes between frequencies all the time. We see simple examples of this in ice ages, pendulum swings from decreasing and increasing earth temperatures which have clear effects on the structures of the earth. Another example is of the seasons. In spring energies lighten up and open up. In winter they close up and retract. Indeed, this movement has profound effects on living entities on earth. The changes are specific and repeated year after year. The same energy changes have effects on the same tissues in the same ways, all the time, every time.

On one hand there is the connection between outside influences and the inner world. Bear in mind that the human being is capable of "paying attention", which allows him to dim the incoming energy messages or to open up to the messages. On the other hand, we have the structure that allows us to learn more about what exactly it is, which of the frequencies are doing what that affects which part of our system. From this we can begin to connect parts of our physical structure to frequencies. This will allow us to determine those parts of the body that get strained by specific frequencies.

The system of life

I found it very interesting when you said our cells are equipped with antennae to pick up information from the outside world, precisely so that the inner world can react to the environment, and that these antennae can be connected or not. Now – as we speak in the middle of lockdown – there is a lot of talk about the dangers of 5G waves. Do we humans have the ability to switch off the antennae of our cells so that we are not affected by anything in particular like this in our environment?

➤ Life is a communication system. There is a constant exchange of information between a great variety of energy fields. Because of everything being made from the same basic information structure, combinations of seven "frequencies", what happens in one part of creation potentially has an influence on the same frequency in any other part. Frequencies are carriers of information, and the frequency relates to the content of that information. We have identified seven different types of information:

1. form
2. movement
3. personal power
4. balance
5. communication
6. intuition
7. knowledge

Each of these is made up of all seven but in different combinations. All energy fields exchange information through the process of interference. Two waves with similar frequencies that come in from certain angles may alter the shape of a wave. This means that that particular bit of information, concerning the content of the frequency, will have shifted slightly as a result of outside interference.

Everything that has been created has a harmonic, a basic frequency that holds the underlying frequencies together. This shows itself to us as a unit. Everything that has a particular shape and a stable form is in balance. It has a harmonic. For example, I can see a range and specific combination of frequencies as a glass, with a specific shape and consistency. The human structure also has a harmonic. Whatever shape it is, it is in balance. Even a body we determine to be misshapen or physically handicapped is in total balance given the information from which it has been constituted. There is a specific balance in every single human life, otherwise it would not keep together. No two are the same. Each one is uniquely constructed and has limited scope before the structure threatens to fall apart, just as a specific sound frequency sound can shatter a champagne glass and break the harmony that held it together.

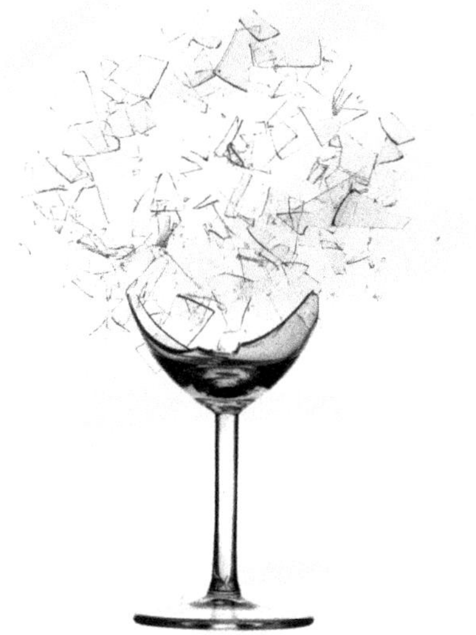

The interference of inner frequencies with frequencies that surround structures will put strain on fixed manifestations of creation. In other words, each human being has been constructed in a very specific way and has a balance that holds the parts together. When that balance gets disturbed through interference from an outside source, stress will be put upon the fixed, created, structure of that life. It is trying to hold on, trying to keep its balance, which is the real struggle for life. And indeed, as we see in nature all around us, survival is about finding our way in the outside environment. Plants and animals alike are searching for food and sustenance. At the same time, they are dodging danger. It is a simple interplay between looking for what they need and avoiding destruction.

What does all of this mean to a human being?

Here is an example. If society puts a lot of emphasis on mobility, frequency 2, then every part of the human body in which frequency 2 has a prominent place will potentially be affected. These could be places in the mobility system, mainly the pelvis, hips and legs. In the sensory system it could be the ears and/or voice and lead to throat problems. In the nervous system it could be the lower back. In the digestive system it could be the gut. It isn't necessarily that all these places will show signs of straining but these are some of the possibilities. Here the relevant questions are:

1. Why will a specific effect show up in one particular area and not in others?
2. Why are some people affected by specific environmental pressures and others are not, or are affected differently?

Cellular antennae

The answers to those questions are provided by one and the same physiological feature, the millions of antennae on the outside of each cell membrane. Each of those antennae is listening for and picking up a specific frequency from the environment. When an antenna gets triggered by a specific vibration it will deliver a signal to the inner workings of the cell and a predetermined response will be activated. This response has been copied from elsewhere by the developing organism. We learn by copying behaviour and our behaviour has been recorded and encoded within the cells. We have an automatic cellular, and therefore also general, response to most more or less "regular" environmental stimulations. This makes life a lot easier and allows more space and time for learning new things quickly.

We can identify two basic groups of antennae related to the jobs that depend upon the information they collect.

The first group is those that are connected to vital reflexes and behaviour patterns, vital in terms of sustaining life. Some of these are genetically determined because the reaction patterns that serve the organism to survive have been established by many previous generations and are recorded and encoded in the DNA. Others are more recent in evolutionary terms and relate to newer reaction patterns required for surviving in a changing environment. Nevertheless, all these antennae are absolutely necessary for the survival of the organism and there is no "willpower" that can switch them off. They are always alert, even when we sleep or are distracted.

The second group brings in information that we require for growing, learning and evolving as individuals and as a species. However, they are not essential for immediate threats to our survival.

The environment is buzzing with information of all kinds and it is impossible for us to notice and pay attention to everything at once. When we observe human senses, we notice that we all observe in different ways. Some of us notice certain things and others notice different things in the same environment. It is no different for our cells. They are unable to take on board all the information out there and it is impossible to "respond" to every little thing. It would also be totally inappropriate. We would never be able to finish a single task because we would be continually interrupted. This means that at any given time there are a number of antennae that are out and active while others have been retracted and switched off. When an antenna is inactive it does not make contact with the information in the environment and that information does not entering the cell. The cell cannot respond to that specific outside information and it is as if that information does not exist.

The activation and inactivation of cellular antennae never stops. We notice a similar system with our senses if we have not heard something *because we weren't paying attention*. When a cell is not paying attention it isn't "hearing" anything. This activation and inactivation is a result of what "the boss" of the organism, the person, wants, requires or demands. *You* decide what antennae are important to you at any given moment in time. Whatever you have decided you need to know, consciously or unconsciously, you will open yourself up to that information. You will allow that information to enter your system. Don't forget that every signal entering the system elicits a response from the metabolism of the cells. What you pay attention to will be important to you. What you don't, doesn't really exist for your system.

Any toxicity in the environment can only affect your health if you open yourself to that information. This was confirmed by a study looking at the negative impact of smoking cigarettes on people's health. It examined the hospital medical records of people with serious lung disorders, put in historical order. Cigarette smoking became a social habit during the industrial revolution and yet a massive peak in lung problems did not occur until the beginning of the major anti-smoking campaigns in the middle of the twentieth century.

That indicates that not all information from our environment affects us. We only have to respond to the information we *choose* to hear. That immediately accounts for the fact that no matter how harsh the outer circumstances might be – an atomic bomb explodes in my city – there will always be people who survive. Perhaps we should pay less attention to what "potentially" makes us ill and start finding out what will keep us healthy. The key lies with the antennae on the cell membrane.

I understand the essence of all this. It makes sense, but at the same time it seems very naïve and idealistic, to think that something will not harm us if we don't pay attention to it. Is it really 100% possible? How much of this has to do with unconscious reasons that we cannot control? Can it apply to anything? What about a poison, vaccine, radiation or injury?

From this perspective, nothing can harm us if we don't want it to. There would be no such thing as "real" and everything would depend on our "point of view", wouldn't it?

➜ I am going to expand on this and make two important points:

1. All cells communicate in this way, but only human cells have a number of antennae that can be switched on and off by someone. This means that most of our reactions to out-side stimuli happen because we open a frequency channel, deploying a specific antenna. Of course, almost all of this happens at an unconscious level and is related to survival in ways we have accepted from we have been told.

2. The main factor in becoming out of balance is an overload of information. This means there is not one cause of a disease but an accumulation of influences.

These two points are really important in understanding and explaining the true disease process at an energetic level. Life is never the same. Circumstances inside the person and outside them are constantly changing. You never arrive at "the same" point again. Understanding this, it becomes obvious that if we want to ensure we are no longer susceptible to illness we must have the ability to withstand becoming imbalanced. However, reaction patterns that are not directly relating to survival have been learned at a very early age, have become automatic and are triggered at an unconscious level.

How can we possibly achieve health if almost all our reactions are governed by unconscious automatic survival reaction patterns or have become automatic?

➤ I will go into detail about this later but first notice that these reaction patterns are constant. "Press the button" and you will always get the same response. Alongside this life keeps changing. A specific reaction pattern I learned when I was a child, one that worked very well then, may no longer be as effective or, even worse, may harm me at a later stage. However, whatever the current circumstances, my system's response to a specific stimulus that triggers a specific antenna, remains the same. When the automated reaction patterns are no longer appropriate for my changed condition my health will decline. All sorts of things go wrong, things connected to a reaction pattern that no longer serves me. Now is time to change it. That is if I want to become healthy again, if I do not want to remain ill. It is absolutely clear that I can only do that by changing the way those cells have always reacted to particular stimuli. I need to recreate the specific reaction the cell has to the specific stimulus. There is no other way. That is the way I need to go to find real and lasting health.

Learning to rewrite unconscious automatic reaction patterns is not as difficult as it may seem, but it takes courage and perseverance. For you to realise what reactions push you out of balance you need to commit to serious self-observation. Whenever you notice you are not feeling well, rewind the clock a little. What has just happened? What are your circumstances? Observe what the situation is like and what your reaction was that has resulted in you feeling bad. Gradually you will be able to recognise patterns: specific circumstances lead to specific reactions which make you feel bad. Stop defending your reaction. Stop finding excuses for your reaction. Simply observe what your reaction is and how it is responsible for how you feel.

Once you know how you respond to that specific situation you need to become alert to both your unconscious reaction and the causal circumstance. When you recognise the circumstance watch out for allowing your system to respond "as you normally do". Choose another response, no matter how ludicrous this may seem to you. Stay alert to recognising when you are responding in the same old way again. Once you realise that then stop it. Do anything you need to in order not to allow the automatic full response to be downloaded. Stop as soon as you notice what your system is doing. Change it to something else. Retract the antenna. When you consistently consciously interfere in an automated programme and you consequently manage to alter the expression of that programme, your system will be getting the message that you no longer want the old response. It will begin to change the way you respond to the same old situation. You have effectively rewritten an unconscious automatic cell programme. Persistence and vigilance is all that is required. Oh yes, and being honest with yourself!

The human body is an organised machine of innumerable parts and all of them, even though they may have different structures, are nevertheless directed towards the same end, which is to distil the humours by which the individual human being lives.

There are two elements of which this admirable microcosm is composed, as well as other non-linear things: matter and movement.

Matter is a mass of innumerable, minute and indivisible parts, to which the Creator has given different forms; and the movement is none other than a mosaic made of all that has been created.

The Creator is he who composes the mixtures; he who sinks and separates things; he who gives and varies forms; and, to put it in a word, the soul of the world, or nature itself.

If he is put into a seed, he gives it life, supplying it with all that matter which it then has to expand according to the three dimensions of its species.

Yesterday and Today.
El mundo engañado por los falsos medicos
Extract from the book

IV

A CURE, A RETURN TO BALANCE

In the previous chapters you have taken us through the creation of mammals and human beings. How should we humans behave in our environment in order to maintain the balance that is so necessary for health?

-❧ Let's simplify the picture. We have a big external world where lots of things are happening, a world of constant change and evolution. Then there has been the creation of a separate entity, a living organism, which occupies a small space closed off from the big world. It is separate and has its own regulatory systems for functioning properly, its own requirements and its own limits within which it needs to remain for staying alive and functioning. Then there are communication channels, "gates" between the outer and inner world. There are different gates through which information can enter or leave the inner world. You might say there is a main entrance, several side entrances, a delivery entrance, a trade entrance, a secret entrance, and so on. It is important is to realise that particular information arrives at specific gates.

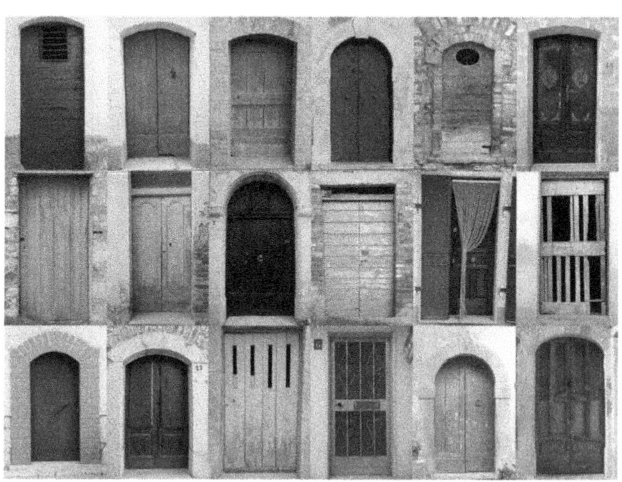

How does the inner system operate?

➤ It requires outside input, outside information to keep the inside flow going. Stagnant energy will decay and rot. People, living organisms, will become ill and may die. Information can only enter the inner world, through the appropriate gate in the fence that separates the inner from the outer world. This can only happen when the owner of the building opens the gate!

Information that does not enter is of no consequence to the inner world. It is as if it doesn't exist. You can't see what you don't want to see. As the saying goes, you can lead a horse to water but you can't make it drink. What stays on the outside does not alter the inside. Unless *you* allow the information to enter, it does not affect your inner world. Once it enters you have an automatic standard way of responding, always the same – until you change it. Consequently, health for an individual is an inner balance that may become disturbed by inappropriate and ineffective inner functioning as a direct result of the influx of information and the way it is dealt with. Which doors we open when and the automatic way we deal with the influx disturbs the inner balance. The duality of life is also embedded within this mechanism: we need energy to flow, so we need to open up. When a fresh input alters what was there before and disturbs the balance, it is the task of the owner of that particular life, to maintain the balance to the best of their ability. There are two basic principles at your disposal:

1. Become aware of which gate you open for which type of information
2. Become aware of your unconscious automatic reaction patterns

You talk about "keeping the inner flow going", which flow do you mean?

➤ The inner flow – movement – to which I refer to is what the Chinese call Chi, Ayurveda calls Prana and Westerners call vital energy.

Everything is energy, and energy is essentially movement. When energy becomes matter, it becomes fixed, and we call that "energy of matter", as opposed to "kinetic energy", "energy of motion". Matter will dissolve again and return to free flow again once "the tension" has been released. All non-living matter is also known as "dead matter". However, all living matter, all organisms, have movement, both internal movement, such as metabolism, and external movement, through changes of position in their environment. Movement can only be seen when energy is flowing through matter, the body.

My body, my castle

A simple way to get to know the body is to compare it with a house with several rooms. Our house has seven rooms and each room has a specific purpose. The bathroom, the bedroom and the kitchen are all rooms, but they are built differently, depending on the function each room has. Furthermore, it must be obvious that, although we have the same rooms in our houses, in each house the rooms have significant differences. We may recognise a room in our neighbour's house as a bathroom because it has certain features we associate with bathrooms, but the specifics of shape, size and layout, may differ greatly from our own bathroom. Each house is unique. Although we are all built in a similar way with the same materials, we all end up different.

Why can't bathrooms all be the same? In different houses they need to be different to function properly. If your bathroom is situated on the north side you may need more heating. If it is small with a little window the window will need to be left open longer to refresh the room. Large baths require more water than small ones. The fact that the rooms are differently constructed means they function differently and are affected differently by circumstances. It is up to the occupant to ensure reaction patterns for optimal functionality in each of the rooms.

This example shows you that there aren't any outside circumstances that are "best" for all buildings, and it is the same for us. There isn't any general health advice that ensures each person functions optimally all the time. What is beneficial to one is detrimental to another. Each owner is responsible for the better or worse functioning of his or her construction. It is up to the owner to respond to changing circumstances in a way that is appropriate for his or her construction.

Let's identify the seven "rooms" and their functions. Within the body there are seven different and separate systems. These are:

- lymphatic system (water system)
- circulation system (blood system)
- feeding system (digestive and breathing system)
- mobility system
- communication system
- nervous system
- glandular system

Of course, each of these rooms, each of these systems, are built from the same materials and the same information, but are different in different people. The building materials are:

- water
- blood
- muscle
- fat
- bone
- nerves
- seeds

Or in terms of information that creates the various building blocks that results in the construction of the different rooms, each with a dominant expression and a particular function, we can list the content of the information as follows:

- Creates the new shape
- Creates balance between history (mother shape) and the present (new shape)
- Creates insight into the distinction between the new individual and the old seed structure
- Creates movement within the new structure
- Creates open exchange between new structure and surroundings
- Creates knowledge about what the new structure means (about life itself)
- Creates the personal strength for becoming a real independent entity

Although this information is used to construct all the "rooms" and therefore the entire structure, there are rooms that contain a larger amount of some information and less of other. This means that changes in that specific information layer will affect certain areas of life more than other areas. In order to easily identify the links between the building blocks, the information layers and the bodily systems we have linked each of them to a figure. The sequence from top to bottom is 1-4-6-2-5-7-3. Each of these has been made up of the same seven layers but in different combinations and, according to our calculations, this results in the following scheme:

1	lymphatic system	mostly 1 and 3	little of 5 and 7
4	circulation system	mostly 4 and 6	little of 5 and 7
6	feeding system	mostly 6 and 4	little of 3 and 7
2	mobility system	mostly 2 and 5 (or 6)	little of 1 and 3
5	communication system	mostly 5 and 7	little of 1 and 3
7	nervous system	mostly 7 and 5	little of 1 and 3
3	glandular system	mostly 3 and 1	little of 5 and 7

It can be seen that when information 1 changes it will affect mostly the lymphatic and the glandular system, whilst information 7 will affect mostly the nervous and the communication system.

This is a simplistic way of representing the basics of life. Each person is a unique construction with rooms that have certain specifics that are unique to that person and each room has a gate that opens onto the environment allowing information to flow between the inside of the construction and the outside. The owner regulates when and how to open and close the gates to their cells and organ systems.

I assume you will talk about when and how to open and close gates, but first, I have some questions about what you are explaining. Where does this theory come from? From ancient medicine? From your own research?

My co-author Erik and I have developed this theory from existing information from different sciences and disciplines. The division of the tissues into seven parts and the seven systems of functioning goes back to Ayurveda, the ancient traditional medicine of India.

What I call gates have been mentioned in the "New Biology", since the 1980s. Then it was discovered that chemicals such as hormones are produced by all the cells of the body, not just the glands. This is the result of frequency stimulation. It was shown that these frequencies are picked up by cells through what they described as antennae. These antennae, when stimulated by the right frequencies, send signals to the inside of the cells. There specific chains of action are produced as a direct result of "picking up the signals". Subsequently, they also showed that DNA reading occurs in a similar way, with the protein coat surrounding the DNA opening and closing depending on the energetic frequencies of the environment.

Through biology, I understand that living organisms function by activating automatic responses in reaction to stimuli received from the environment. From psychology I have learnt that human life involves acquired behavioural patterns, through which the same responses to the same circumstances are always generated automatically.

Why are the systems arranged in that order: 1, 4, 6, 2, 5, 7, 3? Why not 1, 2, 3, 4, 5, 6, 7?

☙ The numbers 1 to 7 relate to the colours of the rainbow, in that order, the frequency bands of visible light. The frequencies follow each other in this order:

1. Red
2. Orange
3. Yellow
4. Green
5. Blue
6. Indigo
7. Violet

In our book *"Why Me? Science and spirituality as inevitable bed partners"* we show that these frequencies repeat themselves over and over again in the Creation of the Universe and in the creation of every living being. The creative process occurs in a set order of frequencies, according to the golden ratio, which happens to be 1-4-6-2-5-7-3.

What does it mean by building with information? What do you mean by "information"?

☙ The building blocks that constitute the physical structure of a body are matter. Matter is condensed energy. Energy is a flow of information. Therefore, the material building blocks of our life are condensed information, fixed information. There are mainly seven different types of information, related to the seven colours and the seven numbers. A frequency means something, and contains certain information about that something.

Frequency 1, contains information about the shape of things.

Frequency 4, about the balance of things.

Frequency 6, about emotions, perceptions and intuitions.

Frequency 2, about movement.

Frequency 5, about communication.

Frequency 7, about learned knowledge.

Frequency 3, about personal power.

In addition, each of these frequencies is formed from the same seven basic frequencies, always in different combinations. This explains the great diversity of life, both in energy and matter.

It would be necessary to go deeper into the building blocks in order to get a proper picture of the precise connections and their implications. When we approach something new for the first time, it can seem very complicated, but soon we get the hang of it and we can untangle the knots without being distracted by the intricacies of the thread.

Gateways

Let's go back to "gates". When and how do we open or close gates? Is it automatic? Is it a reaction? Can we learn to open and close the gates at will?

➥ The gates, their size, position in the room, how easy or difficult they are to open, are all part of the initial construction. They are there from the beginning and have been built as designed for that particular house. As a consequence, each person will have his or her unique gateways to the outside world and their characteristics can't be changed.

The first form of a human being, a completed foetus at 10 or 12 weeks, is going to be fed so it can grow. We can imagine that as "wind" blowing open the gates and filling the rooms, making them expand. Each gate collects information in a way that will enhance the basic structure and future function of that specific room. For instance, the kitchen will use the information to create stuff connected to eating and digesting, while the bathroom mainly uses bits of information relating to enhancing cleanliness and excretion. Depending on what kind of information is available in the outside world, one room may be affected more than another. No information contributes to changes in every room in the same way nor will enlarge all the rooms at the same rate. Specific information ends up in specific places. within the construction.

The environment of a growing new human being contains different elements and different kinds of information. Energetic "nutrition", the stimulation each new human being receives and that is used to enlarge and express each room and therefore the entire construction, is different for each of us. At the same time, the characteristics of every gate in each of the rooms merges with the design of those rooms. It all blends together. This means that none of the gates of a particular room within all those human beings are the same either. Different outside information flowing through differently built gates will shape a room differently. Nature gives us all "bathrooms" but each one is unique.

An important conclusion is that once all the rooms that compose, – your life have – been set out in tissues, organs and systems. You live within that unique structure and each part of that structure will require a unique maintenance strategy. It will operate in a unique way, slightly differently from everyone else. It will have its unique requirements to keep it functional. The characteristics each room exhibits will largely determine what that room will require in order to function at its best. The size and shape of the rooms cannot be altered once the building is finished but you are still able to redecorate and perhaps, with effort, refurbish the rooms.

The original growth process is based on information available in the outside world, on the shape and planned function of the rooms and on the way the gates allow information to enter. Because of these pre-set elements, inflowing information automatically moulds and shapes each room and moves it towards its final look and function. Once the room is completed inflowing information will always have the same effect in that room. The same information entering through the same gate automatically ends up doing the same thing.

When a male foetus becomes a fully grown, stable and predictable adult, he likes his routines and displays characteristic response patterns. He knows what he does and doesn't want and 'strives to get and avoid accordingly. His environment knows his strengths and weaknesses and tries to exploit them. When he and his environment are both are focussed on the same aspects of life at the same time there is harmony between the inner and outer world.

He is happy and his life is peaceful. His house has been perfectly built for that environment.

But what happens when something changes? As everything is always on the move, the outside world changes. Even simple things such as the seasons bring different messages to our doorsteps and your inner needs may change too. There may be times when you spend more time in a particular room. You may require more heat or more movement because you feel you are stiffening up or becoming stifled in some way. Either type of change will be felt as a less than optimal functioning of that room. Since life is all movement and changes happen all the time, it makes perfect sense that living organisms, humans included, have ways to respond to changes in order to minimise negative impact and maximise positive impact.

You said earlier that most of our responses to incoming information are automatic, so how do we change?

🕭 Good question. In principle, there are three ways in which one can influence effects on the inside:

1. Change the outside environment
2. Change the way the gates function
3. Change the automatic response of the inside world

Each method can potentially restore harmony. To some degree we are already equipped to cope with ever-changing lives. The knowledge that nothing stays the same in life indicates that a "bad" situation in the environment will pass. All we need to do is to sit it out for a while. Nature does that. If my environment becomes drier than I need for an optimal function, I automatically recycle more water by shutting down the water outflow through the excretion system. If the environment becomes colder I can open some gates wider to allow excess inner heat to flow more freely or I can close some gates to protect my inner world from freezing, depending on my internal requirements. Although the finished structure is fixed it has a little leeway either side of the harmony point which allows the organism to keep on functioning reasonably well for a while. Inharmonious functioning requires more energy of the entire system and is only sustainable for a period of time before "cracks" within the fixed structure begin to appear. We need to know what to do once the cracks become obvious on the outside, once we become conscious that something isn't quite right and we feel ill.

Cracks within the structure

When you talk about cracks on the outside, do you mean the symptoms of disease?

That's right. We notice when something is wrong because we don't feel good. The system has a built-in mechanism that is always trying to bring it back into balance. It adjusts to changing circumstances, swinging around its balancing point. This is automatic and constant readjustment. The balance it is trying to keep is that which it is used to. That includes things we have learned and have come to accept as "normal". It has always been that way, so we keep it that way. It feels uncomfortable to do anything else. However, as we are also changing, the balance point shifts position over time. The world isn't the same as the one where we grew up and we aren't the same either. That results in tension between the outside world and the inside world, thus upsetting the point of balance.

What do you mean? A tension between the child we were and the adult we are now?

‑❧ No, I mean the tension between the outside world and the inside world. As we grow up, learned behaviour is an adaptation of the inner world to the conditions of the outer world.

This adaptation can take a lot of energy and requires constant effort. Initially, we have that energy and are flexible enough to do it, but as time passes and the situation in the outside world changes, especially in turbulent times such as the ones we live in now, the inner world changes as well. Certain tensions become more and more difficult to sustain. We are getting older! Automatic reaction patterns we have learned up till now – may no longer be the most suitable for dealing with the new outside world. This causes a lot of tension between the inner – automatic reactions – and the outer world that is no longer delivering the old information. This tension manifests in physical functioning. We start to get signals that certain actions or routines are becoming a bit of a problem. For no obvious reason we get new aches and pains or our senses and organs struggle more. Medical practitioners encourage us to look for something that can be blamed, perhaps suggesting "you must have been sleeping awkwardly". We are always looking for something to blame, something we ate, something we have done but, in reality, if it isn't something absolutely outrageous totally outside our usual behaviour, then it truly isn't to blame. The real reason is that nature is telling us the old way is no longer suitable. Now we have signs of being out of balance, being ill. The balance is energetic information from the outer world flowing in to serve the inner world. The two are no longer a perfect match.

As was explained earlier, there are only three elements and therefore only three ways of influencing the existing strained balance:

1. the outer world
2. the gateways
3. the inner world

Only by making alterations to any of these three areas of life can we truly rebalance our lives, become healthy and remove the strain and tension between the inner and outer world. Becoming conscious of something not being right makes us focus in the first instance on the outside world, as the medical profession encourages us to do. It is about "finding the culprit". Who is to blame? It is only, with further stages of personal development that people can open themselves up to the suggestion that there are other, more personal, internal, influences contributing towards imbalance.

Finding the "guilty party"

1. The Outer World

When starting to receive signs of malfunctioning more frequently, we should first look at how we live in order to find what factors are making our life hell. We focus mainly on relationships, work and place of residency. When convinced that one or all are making us ill, we want to change them. If we can, we may feel relieved, released from prison, liberated from the shackles of our old life, and health may restore itself.

Very often, though, we have to be quite brutal in making these changes. You can ask your boss to be nicer to you but if they aren't, your only option is to quit work. In other words, changing our environment isn't only up to us. If your pleas are not heard or are ignored you can choose not to stay in that environment. The environment isn't changing but you are choosing a different environment. You have the freedom, or should realise you have the freedom, to change your environment if you decide it no longer serves you in the best possible way. Whether what you change it into will do a better job remains to be seen and is largely dependent on your judgement. Nature will pull you back, or repeat the entire scenario, if you misjudge things.

If you change your living environment, you change the way your life operates. See it as moving to a different culture and adjusting to a new way of living. If you have chosen a culture that suits you better, you will heal.

2. The Gateways

Each type of information has its own "pathway" into our inner world. The effect on the inner world is a predetermined unconscious reaction that we have learned by copying the way our immediate environment responds to similar impulses. Initially we are overwhelmed by the information entering the newly formed system of the foetus via the mother. The foetus learns what the outside world is like through the unconscious reaction patterns of mother. This sets up basic automatic patterns around survival and danger. After birth, we are able to directly connect with information and the patterning of others in our immediate surroundings. The number and importance of contact people will vary as our life expands from mother, father, siblings and grandparents to teachers, playmates, neighbours, groups, schools and so on.

From this information we pick the reaction patterns that best fit our construction the best and our cells learn to set up fixed responses to incoming impulses in order to be able to operate in the most comfortable way, given who you are and your circumstances.

Let's go back to your question about how we can change the gates if they are all fixed. As youngsters taking our first steps into the adult world, we use what we have learned in order to find our way and to survive. Unconscious reaction patterns rule our emotions, our thinking, our beliefs and our actions. We find ways of surviving in the big world. We do that the only way we know, the way we have learned. Mostly we are not even aware that there are other possible ways of seeing the world and of living a life. The system automatically adjusts to the incoming information to the best of its ability. This is limited like everything in the physical world with its upper and lower limits, extremes beyond which the physical structure threatens to crack. Before it does, the system sends out warning signals about mounting pressure. These signals might be pains, changes in or loss of functionality, irritations or swellings. They may be intermittent or chronic but if they disappear and return it still means that the innate healing properties of the system are inadequate to bring it back to normality. If we continue with the same lines of information coming in and triggering the same responses, the system is bound to break.

As information only enters the system through gateways, information from the outside world that we do not allow to enter the system does not provoke a reaction. Think about radio broadcasting. News informing people of a certain event can be spread via the radio and but if you don't tune the radio to the station giving out this news, you won't be aware of it and it won't affect your mood or behaviour. By simply not allowing your system to "listen" to your environment you avoid being swept away by it.

First, it is good to realise you cannot switch yourself off from all outside information. The system won't allow you to do that. It requires information from your surroundings to give you the best opportunities for survival. That is why we are still alert even when asleep. Some information will always find its way inside.

Second, information comes in from many angles. Information created by humans comes towards us from a great many sources so that it is almost impossible to avoid some of it getting into us.

Thirdly, usually it is only after we receive particular information that we respond with "I really didn't need to know that". By that time, of course, it is already too late and a reaction has already been initiated. Once information enters the system automatic responses are triggered immediately, before our awareness makes contact with the information. This begs the question of how we can alter unconscious patterns if they are always ahead of us.

And another important consequence of the way our reaction patterns, our moods, thoughts and actions, happen is that it is inconsequential where and how they were formed. We do not need to know *why* we respond in a certain manner. All we need to know and concentrate on is *how* to alter it. Knowing why I am as I am, doesn't change who I am. Who I am determines how I function. When the system is signalling that it is struggling to function the way it has always done, it is time to change how I function.

If we want to change what enters our system we need to know how it works, because otherwise we are very likely to become frustrated and disillusioned. The only tool we have for altering anything is our consciousness. As long as we are not aware of something, we do not really know that it exists, so we cannot alter it.

How can we begin to become aware of these automatic mechanisms?

The first thing we might become aware of is a reaction pattern, coupled with a complaint from our system. This is usually the point where the doctor would like you to examine what you have been doing, what you have eaten or anything that may have changed in your life. However, when we are talking about recurrent symptoms or ongoing symptoms it should be obvious that the problem cannot be the outside world. This is when our attention should be turned inward. The evaluation should not be of what we have "done wrong" but rather of observing that the system does not like to act or react this way now, even if it seemed to have been fine for decades. This is the time to observe when my system is giving me this message in relation to my situation. For example, instead of considering I had eaten tomatoes, consider the atmosphere or mood in which I ate the tomatoes. How was I feeling while I was eating? Was I worrying about something? Was I afraid of something? How much pressure was I under?

Before anything else we need to become very aware of the connection between certain "energetic" environments and our reactions. We can begin to recognise the kind of information our systems struggle with and what our habitual reactions are. We can become aware of the sets of circumstances, the different kinds of information that affect us badly.

Once I recognise this connection between specific outside information and reactions to it, I begin working on stopping the unfolding of the automatic reaction pattern my system has been using all my life. Stop allowing yourself to feel what you are feeling, and thinking what you are thinking. Stop it. As soon as you recognise a pattern and become aware of your emotions or thoughts you order your mind to stop it. You refuse to listen to your inner chatter. You refuse to act as you would have done up till now. After increased awareness comes the exercise of stopping the reaction pattern. No thinking about it. No internal discussions. No pro's and con's. Don't react as you have done. Don't react.

As you become better trained in these principles you begin to notice that your mind becomes aware of certain information and what it does to you much earlier in the unfolding pattern. You become very alert to that specific information, or anything resembling it. Then you can stop the automatic reaction sooner and sooner until you are able to almost anticipate it.

You will become expert at reading situations in which it is very likely that that specific information will be generated. You can decide to stop taking any notice. Turn your attention away from the situation, turn it inwardly and close the gate. Switch off the radio receiver. Choose another channel. The information is still all around you, but it no longer has any effect on you, as your mind is not "taking it in". You no longer have to respond to the information because you won't be receiving it.

If by any chance you have been taken by surprise and your alertness did not identify the potential difficulty in the situation, you will immediately become aware of the effect the incoming information has on you. At that stage you will be able to shut the gate quickly. Then spend some time telling your system to stop reacting in that way. It will do so quickly as it understands that message from the many thousands of times you have used it before.

You can stop automatic reaction such as these: It works a bit like this:

- If you believe you are tired during the day because you didn't sleep your ten obligatory hours, or whatever number you think you need, you won't be able to alter your tiredness during the day, simply because your brain "knows" why you are supposed to be tired.

- If you believe your boss is openly displaying your mistakes simply to get you annoyed, you won't be able to feel happy at work because your brain "knows" why you are supposed to be annoyed.

- If you believe you get out of breath easily because your cholesterol level is high, you won't be able to breathe more freely because your brain "knows'" why you are supposed to be breathless.

When certain information is available a "fixed" reaction will manifest. That can't and won't change until you "unfix" it. You need to stop repeating the unconscious cycle between information and reaction that in itself reconfirms what you already know. If you stop saying "See, it happened again, so it must be true!" you can set yourself up to design a new reaction.

When your system is no longer bombarded with information it struggles with, it gets more freedom to explore different pathways. Lots of energy will be saved as the system is no longer fighting to survive. Whatever organs or functions were failing before will restore themselves. The inner natural healing processes of all living cells will keep restoring damage day in day out. You will heal, whatever the illness (and illnesses are a manmade naming game), as soon as the incoming pressure on the system relents. This can happen because your environment changes or your responses to the environment changes. Then there is still a third possibility for restoring health.

3. The Inner World

Truthfully, only when the inner world is no longer a fully automatic mechanism, reacting to all kinds of influences as set up during learning stages from foetus to puberty, can we speak of a balanced health status. Only when the unconscious reaction patterns have been adjusted to a new, well-adapted lifestyle can we feel confident that being healthy has become a "natural" state.

For this to happen we need to be able to change the way we feel, think and act right at the moment when it is occurring. In reality this means that we consciously "choose" what to feel, what to think and how to act. This may be a strange concept but it is only so if we are not really aware of how life works.

The incoming signals have, in the early stages of life, resulted in reaction patterns based on what our environment considered a decent way to survive. We entered the world on our own two feet, armed with relevant skills and tools. We adapted what we did to suit those learned patterns. We did our utmost to respond in the way we had learned, even if it took a great deal of effort and was against our inner nature. It was all we knew and so we did it. We keep doing it until we get signs telling us we are cracking up. That should be the point at which we make significant changes. It is also the point at which society and the medical profession support us in not making any changes.

> When you have learned to select a reaction that best serves you given the circumstances, you will be able to maintain balance. You will not be automatically swept away by the circumstances, nor will you need to securely guard your gates and keep carefully checking what is allowed in and what isn't. You will simply select how to respond, no matter what information has entered your inner world. You can elect not to be angry when someone is abusive towards you or treats you unfairly. You yourself have created the hurt you are feeling as a result of your reaction to that information. Instead, you could elect to be happy, to find it funny, to feel sorry for the person, or to do anything else that takes your fancy. Once you are aware that your emotions and actions are a choice rather than "something you can't help" you have freed yourself from the slavery of unconscious reaction patterns. That freedom ultimately gives you the power to maintain your health yourself.

Our conclusion is that the journey towards empowering and healing yourself happens in three stages. First, awareness is about noticing the influence that the outside world has on how you function and that you can change the inside world. This is followed by the awareness that you don't have to allow all information available in the outside world to enter your inner world and that you can choose what to listen to. Ultimately there is the awareness that you have a choice in how you respond and the fact that you can alter your responses according to your current needs.

This is the journey towards real health that need not be threatened by the fading of your own life energy as part of the natural ageing process. We are not supposed to live forever. Hence, every life will be phased out. However, you have the opportunity to die healthily!

I can't help but wonder whether you yourself have already reached the level you are talking about. Are you able to consciously choose your responses to incoming information from the outside world?

-● Yes, but we can all get to the point of choosing our responses. It's simply a matter of concentration. Understanding how the whole mechanism works allows you to use the system effectively. It just takes practice!

Many believe that to recite well is a necessary consequence of qualifications and an insubstantial virtue of the capirote of penance; whereas, falling sick, they resemble certain foolish young birds that, stimulated by hunger, go about opening their beaks to all the birds that fly about, believing those to be the fathers that bring them food; but what often happens is that they meet the birds of prey that take their lives.

So it is with the sick who are anxious and eager for health, who at the smooth talking beak of the physician give him their pulse, and open their mouths readily to any potion, but these miserable creatures, when they think they are drinking health, unwittingly swallow death.

Yesterday and Today.
El mundo engañado por los falsos medicos
Extract from the book

V

THE ROLE OF INFECTION IN HEALING

Medical science tells us that microbes, bacteria and viruses are constantly stalking us. What we should do is to always protect ourselves from them. When they do attack us and manage to "invade" us, the disease called "infection" occurs. What is the role of so-called "infections" in the context of the "true health" of which we speak in this book?

A good way of illustrating this process is to follow the infectious disease process in its reality, not in the medical version. Medical authorities have busied themselves for two hundred years by ignoring and bringing into disrepute the knowledge that an infection is not caused by an outside agent that penetrates all bodily defences in order to destroy healthy tissue and to make the organism ill. Science has proven irrevocably that the agent comes at the end of the disease process and does not cause the illness. Having clarified this important point, let's talk about how the process we call "infection" works.

First you have to remember that everything is energy and all processes are energetic exchanges. The exchanges are, in this case, between the inner world of a person and the outer world, the surrounding environment. Let's take an extreme example to illustrate a few facts about the infectious process.

Imagine that a major natural disaster has happened in a vast region populated by very poor people who are barely able to survive in the best of circumstances. Say there has been a massive flood from incessant rain, all crops are destroyed, and people have no homes or shelters to protect themselves from the elements. There is no clean water, no drinking water and barely any food. People have lost everything and the future looks worse than bleak. It is hopeless.

Such conditions are known "to cause" outbreaks of cholera and diphtheria, both serious, potential deadly, diseases. These are said to be caused by drinking water that has been infected by faeces and other dead, rotting, materials. In these statements from the medical profession, we already encounter the first scientific problems of microbial theory:

- If faeces and/or rotting matter is contaminating the water with cholera bacteria and/or diphtheria bacteria then those bacteria must already have been present to "contaminate" the water. However, in ordinary human faeces those bacteria cannot be found, nor can they be demonstrated to be present in other rotting matter.

- If the contaminated water is the cause of infections in human beings, then you would expect everybody who has been exposed to become ill with those diseases. *However, the truth is that in every major epidemic only a minority of "exposed" people become ill.*

These are fundamental floors in the infection story the medical professionals teach. They are well aware of these essential shortcomings and make huge efforts to make people ignore them. They focus on details, preferably on details no lay person could disprove, such as specifics about the infective agents and laboratory results. They overlook that life-threatening complications may be due to specific weaknesses in the affected population groups or due to their own approach to the crisis. They overwhelm the media with irrelevant and confusing information about the infective agent and its "erratic and dangerous" behaviour. They attempt to keep people's minds away from more fundamental questions and observations. This is exactly what is happening right now with the coronavirus story. Let us ask ourselves these questions:

- If there are no cholera or diphtheria bacteria present before the disaster, how can they then be responsible for the epidemic?

- If only a small number of exposed people effectively become ill, how can the bacteria they are supposed to have been exposed to be responsible for the disease some of these people display?

Let's get back to energy exchanges. People in their everyday lives are dependent on their environment for survival. If all of a sudden this environment changes and destroys the very things these people require for life, they become sharply aware of the hopeless situation they are in. "How are we going to survive? We need this and we need that, and now it is all gone. What are we to do?" If, what they believe deep in their hearts to be true, which is that "there is nothing they can do", something dramatically changes inside them.

The signals from the environment are that "there is no food or water anymore" and that "life as they have known it is no longer here". In that situation some people become weak and ill, while others do not, same environment, two different reaction patterns, two different ways of responding to the same incoming signals. Some, mainly those who are already weak and have little energy, find it impossible to see a way forward, so they cave in. They stop functioning properly. They are overwhelmed by the changes and capitulate. They see no way of surviving, so they begin to die. They do not allow their minds to find ways of restoring balance in their lives, simply because they do not believe it is possible. For others, finding ways of making survival possible is a major challenge. They allow their minds to look for possible solutions and survive under terrible circumstances because deep inside they refuse to give in. They keep searching for answers to seemingly impossible questions, and they find them.

Are you saying that the people who lose the will to live are the ones who will die of diphtheria and cholera, and that the ones who have enough enthusiasm and energy to survive have a good chance of surviving?

That's right, the people who are "struggling to survive", those who keep themselves busy with how to survive, and who don't worry about whether or not they're going to survive, are the ones who are going to have the best chance of making it. What they do in such a situation is the most important thing. Their actions are a manifestation of their will. What they say doesn't matter. It's what they show, what they produce, what they make real – if you want to put it that way – that is going to manifest in their life.

Do young children and infants who also die from these diseases depend on the state of mind of their parents?

In their case everything depends on their immediate environment, i.e. their parents. Children lose the will to live when their parents lose hope and feel helpless. If their parents don't believe they can make it, what hope is left for a young child? The confidence parents have in their chances for survival is manifested in their own actions, which are perceived by children.

It is no use if, in desperate situations, people say they are "going to fight". In my practice, I have come to the conclusion that the people who keep repeating that they are going to fight and overcome their cancer diagnosis are the ones who die most quickly. The truth is to be found within our own observations. Instead, we have learned to speculate on what is best rather than to observe what our own nature shows us to be best. Experts give us statistical probabilities which we accept as truth. The truth is that life is not a game of chance. Life plainly tells the truth. When you see people die in desperate living conditions it is either because they no longer have the mental strength to make the necessary changes or they have given up because they cannot see a way forward and have given up.

I am very surprised that you say those who repeat that they will fight and overcome the cancer are the ones who die in the shortest time. It has often been said that having a positive attitude and a "will to fight" is very helpful for getting well.

A positive attitude is not only expressed in words. In the case of the cancer patients I am referring to, they give their personal power to the doctor and promise to do everything the doctor tells them so that they can "supposedly" survive. The moment they hand their power over to someone else, they are "losing the battle". They are not focused on the message the disease is giving them, nor are they interested in taking advantage of the opportunity life is offering to make changes and to create a better life. They are simply being "the victims". All they do is sit back and wait whilst following instructions. These are not from their own nature but from an industry set up to "take care" of the situation.

Is what is important not the attitude or what people say, but the real changes they are able to make from our capacity to react in new ways?

➤ Our conditions and messages from the environment are vitally important to how our lives develop, but even more important are the ways that we respond. Your personal response determines the outcome. Even if you cannot see a way forward, it will show itself to you may be your ticket to survival. As they say in the Catholic Church, "Trust in God". You may pray to whatever holy person or divine spirit you like. It will certainly help to keep your mind on the survival track and away from the destruction track. Don't put any "logical" obstacles in your mind's way. Follow your instincts, your natural flow. The only purpose of your natural flow is to keep you alive under all circumstances.

This is how every disease process happens and infectious diseases are no exception. It is not the agent, the bacteria, viruses or fungi, etc. that creates illness. An illness was already present and sometimes produces these agents. The real already existing illness is your response to an outside stimulus, or rather your inability to maintain your inner balance in a forever changing environment.

From this standpoint we no longer have to busy ourselves with any of the particulars of bacteria or viruses or what the medical profession tells us about them. That is all irrelevant, whether or the information is correct. What really counts is how you respond to the way your life is developing and unfolding right now. This has nothing to do with animals or microbes, or even pollution, the warming of the earth, or disturbing electromagnetic frequencies. They may be there, or they may not. They may or may not have a potential disturbing effect upon human life. Everything has a potentially disturbing effect! As long as we can focus on the fact that we have an ability to adapt, instead of taking more and more notice of "detrimental" influences, our minds will find ways forward. We have the ability to adapt, as long as we do not obstruct adaptation by not allowing our mind to keep us alive. We have to stop obstructing our minds by thinking we know better.

Stop thinking about your life and start feeling what it tells you. Forget viruses, bacteria and toxins and start to live, in whatever circumstances you find yourself. Enjoy being alive rather than moaning about your circumstances.

That's easy to say, but how do we avoid obstructing our minds and interfering with the natural process of adaptation?

➤ Let's return to the interaction between the individual's energy and the energy of the environment. They "feed" off each other. They influence each other. The more you open yourself up to those outside energies the more internal influence you will experience. We have the impression that there are thousands of different possible influences.

What chance do we have of being alert enough to "know" what to close the gates against?

➤ We have an impression that there are thousands of possible influences, and that is just what it is, an impression. In reality, there are only seven types of energy that the entire universe has been made out of. Therefore, there can only be seven different types of influences we need to look out for. That simplifies things quite a bit and makes it possible for everyone, with a bit of practice, to identify the kind of energy that disturbs their personal balance. Let's take a closer look at each of them.

I would pay for to have that identified Patrick, although I guess – more than ever – it's not a question of money.

The seven types of external influences

1. Formation/origin

This is about the basic construction of things and that relates to its origins of the construction. In other words, where you are coming from determines the basic shape of your life. Every energy stretches across a spectrum from yin, contracted, to yang, expanded. If the family you come from lives a very concrete, defined life, based on strict principles and guidelines, the structure of your life will tend to have strong bonds with that. As an individual you may have a sense you do not belong in your family because a yin construction does not quite suit you. Then you will already know that at some point you will have to leave your family behind. Physical distance and certainly mental distance will be required. On the other hand, your family may be constructed in a far looser way, where everybody takes care of themselves and nobody really interferes in anybody else's life. They tend to drift apart quite easily early on in adult life, but they maintain a good family bond, from a distance.

The point of this is to notice where the balance is for you as an individual. How does your inner world, your deep needs and requirements, compare with the structure you entered into in this life? When you feel comfortable with the way individuals in your family relate to each other, the principles by which the structure functions and the way the family hierarchy manifests itself, then the influx of a variety of impulses from your environment will most likely be nourishing and supportive in your life too. However, when you feel uncomfortable with parts of the family functioning those same, well-meant, impulses will unbalance you quickly and sometimes seriously. In this case you need to begin factoring in a certain distance from your family, moving your life further and further away from your family in order to find a way of life that suits you better. This may involve moving to a different area, culture or environment. It may involve distancing yourself and your own family from, for instance, the way children "should" be educated or any other firmly held family belief.

In general terms, when you feel unbalanced by the influences of the structure you grew up in, you would do well to worm your way out.

2. Movement

This is about the energy of change. Again, we are looking at a spectrum between yin and yang, between very stable, traditional, holding on to how it has been, and transitional, changeable, bringing in the new. This, of course like all energy groups, has a great variety of ways in which it can be expressed. It may be about changing your living conditions regularly or about travel, but it may also be expressed in a certain rigidity of thinking patterns as opposed to being a dreamer, building castles in the sky all the time. Where does your personal balance lie between the need for stability and the need for freedom? Be aware of the fact that there actually is a balance point for each of us at any given moment in our life. By not recognising, not finding this balance point, we are at risk of swinging from one extreme to the other in a hopeless effort to find it, shooting past it time and time again. Knowing which areas of your life need serious grounding and which need more elbowroom becomes crucial in maintaining a personal healthy balance. You can see the importance of getting to know the inner-you really well. Otherwise, you are very likely to live your life mostly out of balance and this is the cause of all diseases. It is crucial to ask yourself which parts of your life require a stable footing and which parts are vital for you for having lots of freedom. Then arrange your immediate environment to suit your needs. Choose the kind of job that fits your life. Choose the kind of partner who fits your life. Choose the place and manner in which you want to live to suit your inner requirements. Some parts of your life will require a lot of movement, lots of changes, and some parts will require very little.

3. Personal power

This energy is about inner strength. Again, think about a spectrum reaching from yin to yang, from being inflexible, stubborn, immovable (and that is where one person's power lies) to being very flexible, adaptable and difficult to corner (another type of personal power). Each of these extremes does have personal power but only for a specific personality. Each would do well to maintain a life in which they are the most powerful person they can be. However, the "measurement" of someone's inner personal power relates directly to the opposing power of 'their environment. In order to live a balanced inner life in an environment that does not pressurise them much (some call that an "easy life"), someone does not need an awful lot of self-empowerment. The more the outside pressure increases the more pressure there is on the inner environment of the person to "fight back" or, more precisely, to resist being crushed to death.

How much inner strength is required depends on the oppressive power of the environment. If there is much oppressive power, we need to keep our gates rather more closed than open.

The other consideration is which aspects of life are mainly in the firing line of the outside world, which aspects of life are being pressurised most and which specific areas you, as an individual, struggle with. To maintain your inner balance, you need to know yourself pretty well. You need to know your strengths and weaknesses and you need to practise protecting areas of weakness. Protection means keeping the gates firmly closed, not allowing too much of that kind of information to enter your system.

How much is too much?

🍵 It is too much when you feel you can't be yourself anymore, when you feel you are being smothered, can't breathe or feel very tired. As with all these aspects, overstimulation from the outside requires closing gates. You may, in the long run, need to change your environment. Under-stimulation requires searching for more appropriate impulses in order to challenge your system in positive ways. In the long run this may also require a change of environment.

4. Balance

This is about balancing the flow of your energies between how much you give and how much you receive. Within the human race there is the entire spectrum from people who are best balanced when they are constantly giving to others to people who are best balanced when they are constantly receiving. The only "good" or "bad" one can consider here is the effect the giving and receiving has on your own life. Creating a "good" feeling when we give is not the same as being balanced. Giving more than you can spare devalues your life. Taking more than you need devalues your life too, in the sense that you become weaker and more and more dependent. As an analogy, if you drink more alcohol than your system requires you become dependent upon receiving it.

Find the balance between giving and receiving. For most of us, balance begins by learning how to receive, without thinking you have to give enough back in order to not feel guilty about having been given something. It is also important to learn in which aspects of life you have abundance, and can therefore give more, and in which aspects you should not give anything, simply because what you have you need for your own survival. We need to know what is truly required for survival, rather than what we think we require from a perspective of fear and lack.

In order to find a balance between what you give and receive it is crucial to know the state of your inner being. What skills and strengths do you have more than enough of and which ones are in short supply? At the same time, what are the limits of what you are able to give at that moment in time? To maintain balance you need to readjust all the time. Let what you give always reflect the abundance you feel in your life. Let what you receive always be a gift to your life.

5. Communication

This is the energy of expression. The spectrum ranges from intro-version to extroversion, but we also need to consider the various aspects of communication and expression. It isn't just about words but about all the senses. It is about expression on all levels, in which every part of the body has a role to play. If you and your environment are not expressing much of your inner activity then that may result in a balanced life for you. Equally, if both you and your environment are extremely expressive that may result in a well-balanced inner state for you. Any other combination, however, will disturb that balance. If your environment is very loud and aggressive in its expressions and you are not, you need to either become very loud (if that is your true nature!) or, more likely, you will need to look for different living conditions. If you are very loud and expressive and your environment is not, chances are that at some point you will get kicked out. In that case, for your own balance in life it would be good to find different ways to express yourself adequately.

The strength of the way we express ourselves is one part but the other is the various *ways* that we can express ourselves. This society favours auditory and visual expression. Over the years this has grown into shouting matches of sounds and colours. Communication happens through all the senses, so we can learn to be more expressive, or less expressive in other ways, always balancing our expression with the ways our particular environment communicates. Communication from the environment is quite different in inner cities and in the countryside. Communication from the human environment has become quite different from communication from nature. Again, you can close the gate for the kind of expressions that disturb your inner balance and open it whenever the intensity of communication becomes disturbing. In the long run, if closing and guarding the gate constantly requires too much energy, it might be necessary to seek a different environment.

6. Intuition

One could see these energies as the more subtle parts of communication. These energies connect to deeper elements of our being.

There is the "sense" of being followed or being watched. and the sensing of something not being right. There is an entire spectrum amongst human beings, from yin, very solid and not very subtle, to yang, being extremely sensitive to any slight change in the environment. Depending on the make-up of an individual one can be in balance in either situation.

A person who has very little intuitive sensations (yin) is not doomed to never have a sense of "what is right". This person may, when well-balanced, still make intuitive decisions without being aware of a "sense "of what is right. Such a person may use the expression "I just know", without any sense of where that came from. On the other hand, a very sensitive but well-balanced person will not necessarily be disturbed and pushed out of balance by every single sensation. They may be able to prioritise impulses relevant at that moment. When someone is out of balance it is more likely that they will become disturbed and may even suffer physical signs of imbalances, i.e. diseases, as a direct result of taking in, and allowing the system to respond to, every single awareness that reaches their consciousness. This hypersensitivity, when it unbalances the system, can make a balanced life almost impossible to sustain.

Closing the gates on impulses that might create an imbalance is a clear and workable option for maintaining balance. Look away. Focus your mind on something else. Do not take notice of every sensation. Close the gate. In extreme situations you might need to move to an area of low stimulus. Take into account that human society has become an environment of overstimulation with too many impulses entering our systems. Going to an environment that connects more directly to the roots of the human being, nature itself, can do wonders to restore that balance. Even so, in the first place I would recommend training your mind to close your gates when necessary, in order to protect the balance of your inner world.

7. Conscious Knowledge

This involves the way we accumulate knowledge. The yang part of the spectrum is logic, thinking and analysing. The yin part involves feelings and sensations. Both parts are an efficient way to gain and retain knowledge. Some people know what to do because their mind follows set rules to reach the end result, while another person's mind may reach the same goal by recollecting sensations. Some retain the code to their smart phone by remembering a sequence of numbers. Others remember it by moving a finger over the keyboard.

In order to keep the function of your nervous system in balance you need to know what kind of knowledge you accumulate and retain via what route. Again, there is no "right" or "wrong" way of learning in general. There is, however, a right and wrong way of learning for each individual. In a world that has overemphasized logical learning and only seems to appreciate logical learning, enormous pressure has been put upon people who learn in a different way. They become unstable. Some are being pushed back into their own inner world and shutting the door to their outside world. Others push themselves into the outside world and show destructive behaviour in order to divert attention away from their weaknesses from having been made to gain knowledge in ways that are inappropriate for them.

It is good for us to get to know ourselves really well, to know how we handle information, create knowledge and retain knowledge. If you lean towards the logical side you need to satisfy that tendency. At times this may shutting the gate on airy-fairy impulses but others may have decided you are living in a too logical world. They may feel you need to get out more and talk to the trees, feeling the energy flow through the branches and sensing whether the tree is healthy or not. On the other hand, if you have a more sensitive nature and you connect with information in a different way, you may need to stop allowing yourself too much logical input and to shut the gate to logic at times.

Each of us needs to know how much yin and yang information is required and what is needed so we can maintain our particular inner balance. You may find that, for instance for building a shed, you need to rely on mathematics and measurements, but when it comes to creating a garden much of what you do does not involve any logic, book knowledge.

There you have it. That is how we find balance!

Right now, this may all seem a bit much but, in all fairness, it really isn't. The reason why it may appear to be an almost impossible task is that most of us have been moved so far away from our natural balance that we have lost connection to natural alarm signals. We have lost the connection to who we truly are.

How do you start repairing yourself?

➤ Begin by getting to know yourself. Stop telling yourself what you need, who you are and what makes you tick. Observe how your system responds when you expose yourself to certain situations, when you allow specific information to enter your system. Observe. Don't jump to conclusions. Just observe. You will soon start noticing that there are differences in your responses where you were convinced there had been uniformity. Soon you will get to know when you respond this way and when that way. Knowledge about yourself that you gain from exercising this way will quickly enable you to see what you need to do to straighten what might have been crooked all your life. Only from inner observation will you be able to balance your life.

Be aware that the seven areas of life, the seven types of energies, are the basic building blocks of all that exists in the universe. That means that endless combinations of these are responsible for all of creation. In human terms it means that every one of those areas has been made up of all seven energies, for each of us in different combinations. This means you need to observe in which area you experience an unsettled feeling. For example, if you find you are completely losing your personal strength (3) at times, keep observing and you will find out exactly what it is that zaps your strength. For instance, you may find out that it happens when your environment forcefully communicates, aggressively expressing (5), itself. It may be that this happens when your environment demands pure strong logical thinking (7). That specifies the circumstances and thereby defines the type of gate you need to guard heavily.

Remember, there is no type of personality or human construction that is better than any other. They each have restrictions (because every incarnation is for learning specific lessons). You have the tools to meet the demands of your life and someone else is equipped with tools that suit their life. The only thing you need to learn is everything there is to know about your own life.

Every day you can learn more. With every exercise, every effort you make, you get to know more about your personal life, about how it is for *you* and how it needs to be. Once you begin to control the gates of your inner city, forbidden to anyone else, you start to realise that only you hold the keys to your happiness, to the balance in your life.

You determine what your life is like and if and when you become ill. This is because illness is an imbalance, and you control the balance of your life. You don't need to control your environment. You do need to control your response to your environment. You do need to ensure your response supports your system. You do need to ensure you serve your system, and your system only. Too little of something creates an imbalance, just as too much creates an imbalance.

Getting it right for you depends on getting to know yourself, getting to know the balance of weaknesses and strengths in all departments of life. Now you know that there aren't that many departments – just seven!

Where do microorganisms come from?

It is curious that the subject of infections has led us to talk about adaptive processes and these seven areas of life. Let's return for now to a common thread, germs. You say that microbes appear at the end of a disease. What is the reason for their presence? How should we act in the short term? While I am having a cholera infection it would be difficult to work on my inner balance.

Microorganisms, such as bacteria, appear in diseased tissue when there is so much cellular debris that a bonfire, an inflammation, is not enough to burn all of it. As is the case with all waste everywhere, living things will appear that feed on it. These microorganisms will feed on the waste of the diseased tissue until they run out of food. At that point, the organisms will disappear and will never be seen again.

Thus, the immediate reaction to a perceived disease should be twofold. Firstly, any fire must be stoked. When there is local heat or fever we must add more heat, because the hotter the fire, the more effective the combustion process will be. Secondly, we must stop dispersing the energy in other directions than towards the disease, the fire itself. This means it is a good idea to stop eating, to stop working and to rest completely. With any acute infection, diagnosed or undiagnosed, you have to take sick leave. You must stay in bed. Sleep and rest. You don't eat, you just drink small sips of herbal teas or warm water, with a little lemon if you like. Let the illness run its course. While it does, do not rob your system of energy through mental fantasies. Stop thinking about and rethinking what you should do. The answer is always the same: nothing. The most effective and quickest way out of an infection is "to do nothing", literally. Does this shed some light on what to do when we have an infection?

It makes it very clear. These simple tips – don't do anything, rest, don't eat, don't fantasise – do they work for all illnesses? For cancer as well?

All diseases come from the same imbalance, whatever the cause of that imbalance. Rectifying the imbalance is healing. This applies to all diseases, including, yes, cancer.

The fallacious theory of microbes

Where does the theory of infection, which argues that the origin of disease is an external agent, come from?

Let's take more than a glance at the origin of microbial infection theory and emphasise that it is just that – a theory.

Everything always starts somewhere, and chronic infections are no different. Doctors observed that sometimes tissues began to rot, with cellular structure disintegrating, and that subsequently people became ill, sometimes seriously, even in danger of losing their lives. This process was observed both in wounds on the surface of the body, as well as in internal organs and tissues. It was proposed that living organisms, invisible to the naked eye, were responsible for this, formulating a scientific theory and thereby establishing what was *believed* to be responsible for this. An external agent was said to penetrate the outer body defences and to interfere with the normal functioning of the cells and the body, making them sick, with possible cell death as a result. If enough cells died, the person's life was in danger. If you think about it, it seems a plausible idea when there is an open wound. In wounds, it was obvious that the outer lining of the body was already broken and that it would be easy for "small invisible creature" to settle in the debris caused by the trauma. However, they extended this idea to other parts of the body which were still intact in their structure at the time they were supposedly penetrated by that organism. That indicated healthy, undisturbed tissue being broken down by invisible creatures. These unknown organisms were assumed to have special powers, including bypassing the body's normal defences, entering the inner world, traveling to specific locations and initiating local tissue destruction.

Medical researchers called these organisms bacteria and decided they were the cause of infections. The medical profession therefore decided that infectious diseases were caused by the infiltration of foreign living organisms into the human body. That was the scientific theory.

The main argument for this was the fact that bacteria could be seen under the microscope. Apparently, not only did these minute creatures exist, but they were also found in abundance in diseased tissues. Their presence there led the profession to assert that these microbes were responsible for the devastation seen in the diseased tissues, since in healthy tissues they were not found, or only present in very small quantities. The mere fact of their presence made them look guilty, so they must be guilty. It was a convenient way of closing the case and putting the matter to rest. The medical profession had found its enemy and was now ready to fight him.

But it is in fighting an enemy that one gets to know one's opponent better as the fight drags on. Has this been the case in the history of bacteria as the supposed culprit of infections?

In the first half of the 19th century, two important events shaped the medical profession in ways that still shape it to the present day. Initially, there were scientific studies that dismissed the theory that bacteria seen inside diseased tissues came from outside. Various experiments, repeated many times in various university laboratories, proved that the existence of bacteria in diseased tissues was a natural phenomenon of the disease itself. It was shown that these bacteria arose from inside the diseased tissue as a direct result of the disease itself and that it was not an invasion of any kind. In other words, bacteria were present, but they were not the cause of the disease. The disease existed before and, in some cases, bacteria arose from the debris caused by the disease.

Scientific evidence does not support the theory that bacteria cause infections. Scientific evidence has demonstrated that bacteria occur as a result of disease and are not responsible for causing it. The scientific theory that bacteria cause infections has been exposed as being totally false.

Around the same time, in trying to establish a causal link between a possible disease factor and the disease itself, the medical profession struggled to find a protocol that could determine cause and effect. Professor Koch wrote four postulates accepted by the scientific world establishing a causal link between the presence of a living microscopic organism and a specific disease. Although these postulates are still valid and scientifically sound, even Professor Koch himself turned away from them and began to downplay their importance, because he could not find a single causal link between organism and disease. Koch's postulates quickly became a footnote in the medical history books, and, to this day, no one has ever been able to establish a causal relationship proving that any bacterium is the cause of any specific disease. When you claim to have found a solid method that separates the guilty from the innocent, but you are unable to establish a single guilty verdict. it seems to be easier to maintain a falsity than to acknowledge your own error. From then on, you can continue with the scam.

At the time investors chose to ignore the scientific community and to stick with the story of invasions of small pathogenic organisms infiltrating and destroying human tissue. They supported the theory promoted by Louis Pasteur. He had said that in order to protect ourselves from disease we would have to fight against these organisms that live all around us. Killing them all, the more the better, seemed like a great idea, as was finding a way for human beings to become "immune" to such barbaric invasions. For this an extensive immunisation programme was devised and, of course, vaccines were developed, tailor-made against each of the known bacteria. The manufacturing of vaccines became a priority mission for the medical industry. Within a few decades vaccines became the "flagship product", promoted as "preventive medicine".

Science versus medical science

From that point in history, the term "medical science" began to be used, a clear distinction from the term "science", which suggests that there is another type of science that is going to take care of our health, a branch external to science itself. Perhaps it is time to mention that the very idea of there being two separate types of science (apart from good science and bad science!) and that the two can arrive at contradictory results, is simply stupid. It would be like saying everything in life has one valid factual explanation, but as soon as we talk about aspects of health in life, the basic rules change.

Surely the truth will have to become victorious over the lie at some point?

-❧ One of the first problems medical theory has to face is the fact that in many infectious diseases it is not even possible to demonstrate the presence of any of the microorganisms, blamed for the disease. Faced with the basic premise that *all* infections must be caused by the invasion of a microorganism, their explanation was a simple one. In such cases, the organisms were said to be so small that they could not be seen. Completely ignoring the fact that science had already proven their theory to be inaccurate, the medical authorities decided to put a new twist on the bizarre story of barbarian invasions by inventing a new "invisible" infectious agent, the virus. Then they postulated that viruses were responsible for such infections and announced that, one day, they would find them. The lie could then be perpetuated a little longer as nobody could prove them wrong. Nobody has any material to work with as "viruses" are invisible.

But they finally found them! Of course, huge sums of money were poured into medical research to find this elusive disease-causing "microbe". Many theories were posted about the whereabouts and morphology of viruses and new research methods were devised, all to find pathogens and invisible agents that had already been predicted. With the advent of the electron microscope in the early 1930s they could finally "see" the culprit. Truth be told, what they saw were tiny specks in and around the cells. These they quickly claimed as the elusive "viruses". That could only be what they had been looking for so long.

Since the idea of demonstrating a causal relationship between a so-called pathogen and a specific disease is crucial to the concept of infectious diseases, and given that up till that time, and beyond, no one in the medical profession had found such a link, it must seem strange that no attempt was made to relate the image obtained under the microscope to the physiology of the disease. First the culprit was named and then anything that appeared in the cellular area in conjunction with an infectious process, had to be "it". The medical profession, medical science, did not prove at any time that what it had found really matched the characteristics attributed to the causative agent of the disease. Does what you see in a photograph reveal what it is said to be able to do? It doesn't matter. They used a much simpler method to determine their truth: "We've found something, so that must be it!"

Now I understand what you are saying about there being good and bad science.

-❧ The medical profession decided at that point to separate the study of these extremely tiny entities from clinical practice. A speciality was created, virology, which deals not with patients, but with viruses inside cells and all kinds of cellular debris. The "virus specialist" is shut in a laboratory, far away from any clinical environment and patient, to immerse himself in the virtual world of the invisible.

According to medical science, viruses are supposed to transmit diseases. Surely, they had to study how transmission or infection occurs?

❧ Listen and don't lose any of the details relating to the supposed transmission of infections. According to medical authorities, there has to be physical contact between an infected area, where the infectious agent is present, and the person who becomes ill as a result of that contact. But medical science is not always able to detect the supposed source of an infection. They solve the problem with the stroke of a pen by assuming that someone may have picked up the infectious agent a long time ago and that the agent has somehow survived inside the body of the infected person without causing any problems. At a certain time, in circumstances unknown, that agent comes back to life, or should we say "activates" itself, and then infection manifests itself. This invents the mysterious healthy and asymptomatic carrier. It cannot be proven but, more importantly, it cannot be disproven. Now they can say, when they cannot locate the source of infection because there has been no direct contact with an infected person or area, that you may have been infected by a healthy carrier. This "small detail" eliminates the hassle of having to identify the source of infection.

As if that were not enough, the possibility that these infectious agents can be transported was introduced. From that premise it was no longer necessary to have direct contact with an infected person. You may have "picked up" the infection through the air, water or a solid surface. This could be the ground or whatever they want to it to be. As bacteria exist everywhere they could demonstrate their presence anywhere they liked. They were already able to use the mere presence of bacteria as a cause and as the origin of any infectious process. The transfer theory is impossible to disprove, since science has truly established that all life on earth depends on the existence of living organisms such as bacteria, fungi and parasites. This means that their presence can always be demonstrated in the vicinity of people who fall ill.

If you simply assume, as medical authorities do, that being present is tantamount to being guilty, you have found the solution to the question "who is to blame", a solution no one can refute. Since, from the outset, the medical authorities have evaded the need to establish a causal relationship, as well as turning a deaf ear to accepted scientific practices, none of them are able, any longer, to acknowledge the errors they made. They are unable to recognise the lack of an essential requirement which, in their view, was never an essential requirement. They are unable to recognise the intrinsic conflict in the idea of an infectious agent attacking from the outside and that such an infectious agent is, at the same time, an essential part of the structure of life. They do not acknowledge this contradiction. They have been told in their university education that these two things are not the same thing. Welcome to the cognitive dissonance of an entire profession.

Is there any evidence that medical authorities are completely wrong about how infectious diseases are spread?

Apart from the fact that the presence of a microbe in a diseased tissue is not by itself proof it is the cause of the disease, we encounter even bigger problems when it comes to viruses.

The actual information available about the characteristics of viruses includes that these entities are not alive. There is a huge difference between viruses and living organisms such as fungi and bacteria:

- The structure of a virus is of such simplicity that there are no internal organelles, which means that viruses have no metabolism and are unable to metabolise anything. They are incapable of doing anything. This confirms that a virus is not a living organism.

- A virus is only "active" inside a living cell, it can only "survive" inside a living cell. How can a thing that is not alive have an activity and be "active" inside a living cell when it has been clearly demonstrated that it does not have that capacity? How, in any case, can an entity that is not alive survive when it is not alive?

- It is said that the small, single-stranded genetic sequence of a virus will infiltrate a cell's DNA and "force" it to produce copies of the virus. But how it is able to do that is never mentioned, only that it does. The infected cell is supposed to be forced to produce copies of the virus until it is completely filled with copies of the original and explodes, spilling its contents all around it, infecting neighbouring cells and causing the disease to spread.

Only a few pictures have been taken with electron microscopes, but the existence of viruses is impossible to prove in clinical settings. There is no scientific evidence of the actual activity of a virus inside a cell, nor of the behaviour of a virus outside of a cell. We do not have any "live" video of viruses moving or performing activities. To fill these gaps, medical authorities simply borrow the story of bacterial infection they themselves originated without evidence. This is nicely reinforced by the fact that people have already accepted the argument that "it must be true because no one has been able to disprove it". Repeat a lie often enough and with sufficient authority and it will become an accepted truth.

What comes from this view of microorganisms is that:

- If the presence of infectious agents, even invisible ones, means that they are responsible for an infectious disease,

- if infectious agents can mutate from good and helpful to bad and destructive,

- if infectious agents can be transferred by water, air and surfaces – such as soil,

- if infectious agents can be present in a latent state inside a healthy individual, who then becomes an unwitting spreader of disease, then you have built the foundation upon which you can manoeuvre in all directions to "explain" everything, without having to prove anything at all.

- You stick to your theory. You can even expand on that unproven theory. You can add exceptions to an extension of the unproven theory. You dismiss comments or questions such as: "Don't you think it is possible that…?"

Now medical authorities have relieved themselves of the burden of proving the theory and have put the onus of disproving it onto "anyone opposing it", they feel confident enough to declare it as absolute truth. They can use any of their hypotheses to develop new assumptions, believing that their theory constitutes a sound basis from which to work.

The lack of truth in disease transmission

A stage in the process infection is the so-called "incubation period", the time between being "infected" and the onset of the disease. How does the medical profession fit this into their theory?

➥ Early in its history, medical science proposed a different incubation period for each infection, varying from five days to two weeks. According to the medical authorities, this is the period from the time the theoretical external invader infiltrates a new victim to the time they begins to show symptoms of the disease. During this incubation period the attacker finds a suitable place in the body where it can take refuge, multiply and use the cells' resources to feed itself, and all its comrades. This process, supposedly, drives the cells to death. That is when what they call "an infection" manifests itself.

At the same time, the medical profession has established that an infection has to manifest itself before it can become contagious, a new source of infection. In other words, you can't spread invading microorganisms around to others until your own tissues have been damaged by the infection. Also, in order for another person to be infected, there has to have been direct contact with infected material from someone. The mere fact of being in their presence was not sufficient for infection or transmission to occur. Close contact was essential. But…

- Observation of the foci of infection and their contacts has shown that infections could not be linked to close contact with infected material

- Observation of the possible causes of infection has shown that there was no link between the presence of the infectious agent and the disease

- Observation of the speed with which an infection seemed to spread through the population has clearly shown that, although the idea of an incubation period is essential to the theory, the time lag was not being respected by nature

At this juncture, a logical and scientific approach to the theory of infection would have been to conclude that there was no evidence for continuing to defend it.

However, instead, medical authorities changed their postulates and decided that infectious agents must "obviously" be transported, for example through air, soil and in microdroplets of water. Their story expands into doorknobs, money, toothbrushes, towels, etc. so that our invader could spread over long distances, far from the original source of infection. Again, our friends, as has become their habit, have not tried to prove such a claim. They have left it to the rest of us to disprove it. Fortunately for them, no one has bothered to do so. By that time, medical science had already drawn its conclusions about the validity of the externally caused infection theory. From a truly scientific perspective it was null and void, incorrect and unworthy of further attention. Since an entire construct based on erroneous assumptions has by definition no scientific meaning it is utter nonsense.

If this is all solemn nonsense, then what is the value of the various diagnostic methods the medical profession use to "prove" someone is suffering from a viral infection?

What medical science has accepted as common practice to test for the presence of a virus is:

1. The identification of a small sequence of DNA/RNA sequence without knowing where it comes from. This DNA is replicated several times in a laboratory so that it can then be found, in large quantities. among cellular debris. No amount of a DNA sequence can be linked to a specific invader, nor to any particular activity such as causing a disease.
2. The measurement of a high level of antibodies in the blood as "proof" of an immune response of the body, assumed to be triggered by and directed to the unidentified invader, the virus they claim that is causing the disease. However no scientific link between a specific antibody and a specific "invading" agent of any type can be found. Antibodies are not found to be specific to any particular disease or infectious agent.
3. The measurement of a high level of specific cells in the blood as proof of an immune response of the organism, which is assumed, to be against the unidentified invader, which would have to be the virus that is said to be causing the disease. However, no connection between the type of blood cells and the quantity of those cells in the blood has been scientifically established, nor has there been any connection with an "invader" of any kind. In other words, no

level of white blood cells is specific to any disease or infectious agent.

For the medical profession, any one of its diagnostic tests will serve, not only for the identification and confirmation of which disease you are suffering from, but also to demonstrate that the causative agent of that disease is present. The tests work both ways: a virus, and only a virus, gives you a positive test result, and a positive test result tells you which virus it is. I call this, at the very least, "manipulative science".

How is it that, when medicine has all this difficulty, so many have applied themselves to the same study?

For, being divided into various sects, some have laboured in one way, others in another; but the attempt of all being equally vain, it is clear how arduous the study of true medicine is.

Three were those who, among all the other sects, acquired some applause from the ancients, but it has already been acknowledged that they were all very far from that essence which alone constitutes a good physician; and that is, "To cure safely, speedily and agreeably".

Yesterday and Today.
El mundo engañado por los falsos medicos
Extract from the book

VI
ON VIRUSES AND OTHER TALL STORIES

Patrick, since we have been talking about viruses and bacteria, I think there are many questions that have not yet been adequately answered in relation to the supposed coronavirus pandemic which started in 2020. What is your position on the existence of the coronavirus?

Does it exist? Does it not exist? Is it a lie? Was there a real reason to declare a pandemic?

For human beings, "exist" often means that something has been proven to be present in a physical way. We need to measure it or be able to see it. The existence of bacteria was only confirmed when they were seen under a microscope. Similarly, the existence of energies will only be accepted once they can be measured. This is also the reason why many human beings, including scientists (the intelligent ones), are reluctant to accept the concept of God.

If we want to ask about the existence of coronaviruses, which are a type within the larger concept of "viruses", we must first address the question of the existence of viruses in general. If you ask me if a "virus" has ever been seen, the answer is yes. "Virus" is, in fact, the name given to a small, encapsulated bubble seen in the electron microscopic image of a cell. This image is obtained after a long and difficult process of preparing a very thin sheet of living matter which has had to be killed in order to examine it under an electron microscope. Therefore, the image obtained has no movement and is in black and white. However, some of the small, encapsulated particles seen inside the cell, at the edge of the cell and outside the cell (information gathered from many photographs) have been called "viruses". This means that viruses exist, because we have pointed at something and we have given it a name.

However, the significance of viruses, what they do and how they work, are separate matters from their mere existence. If I show you images of a figure, either standing in the hallway of a house or leaning against the front of a house, or outside in front of the house, and I say to you, "this is a man", then that figure is a man. From now on you will recognise that figure as that of a man. The existence of "man" is real because I perceived something and called it "man". When I later tell you a man just like that steals, burns and destroys, and furthermore I support what I tell you with pictures of a man inside a bank, next to ruins and in front of the burning city of Rome, you may want to believe me. Does, however, the mere presence of that man in certain places, and at certain moments in time, really make him the kind of character I am presenting? This is not the right way, the scientific way, to go. The best thing to do is to gather the information science has been able to obtain about viruses and their behaviour and to draw conclusions from that.

First of all, the physical structure of a virus can most easily be described as a piece of genetic material (DNA or RNA) encapsulated in a single membrane pocket. Or, in other words, it is a small bag containing a short sequence of genetic code. Surprisingly, inside that pocket there are no other organised structures, such as an energy production system, a circulation system or a nervous system. Indeed, scientists have determined categorically that viruses "do not feed, excrete or move". For all intents and purposes, they are not alive. They cannot replicate on their own. They cannot multiply as they have only a single strand of genetic code and are said "to use" the metabolism of host cells to reproduce. Consequently, they are said not to be "alive" because they cannot perform any of the vital functions that constitute life.

It is also said that this small inert bubble can make its way through the mucous membranes of our respiratory system and digestive systems. Some doctors even claim it can find its way in via our eyes, bypassing our "anti-invasion system", whatever that means. Apparently, they then camouflage themselves in order not to be detected in the bloodstream, again completely outwitting our immune system's "patrol cells". We are told that once they find the right organ they manage to penetrate the highly protected three-layered cell membrane without the cell giving the slightest indication that anything might be wrong. Once inside the cytoplasm of the cell and the heavily protected nucleus of the cell they still have no role to play because they don't do anything. They can't do anything. They have no metabolism. They do not "function "in any way, shape or form. But despite this deficiency we are told about the "heroic journey" that every virus makes through the internal machinery of the cell, how it makes its way through another membrane, and through another also heavily protected one, into the nucleus of the cell, into the cell's control chamber.

Here "the little virus dwarf" is confronted by a gigantic structure with complex genetic coding like the internal layout of a computer's memory. The internal coding of the virus can be compared to approximately three or four words from the complete works of Tolstoy. Yet we are told that these three or four "words" are able to strategically sneak into the full text, the genetic code of the cell, supposedly with the result that all cellular metabolism is now at the service of the virus. A few words have managed to change the entire story! A virus is supposed to force the cell to produce nothing but more viruses. Quite a feat for a small bag containing only a few genetic codes and without any ability to do anything at all, no capacity to perform any kind of action! Quite a feat, don't you think?

Exosomes

Recently more and more researchers and professors have been renaming viruses as exosomes. They want to create a different image of these particles from the one they have historically been taught. There are reasons for this. It is typical of human history. First we saw sharks only as indiscriminate killers, only to find out later that this was a complete mistake.

What do scientists mean when they refer to something as an "exosome"? Exosomes are small particles that appear inside cells, particularly in cells that have trouble functioning in a normal way.

When these exosomes increase in number, they are pushed to the outer layer of the cell, the membrane, and from there the cell excretes them. The cell may or may not recover from this, but it is quite clear that these exosomes originate from inside diseased cells and are excreted by the cells themselves. What do exosomes consist of? A simple membrane that encapsulates a small piece of genetic code. Sounds familiar? Instead of the complicated and hazardous journey from our surroundings into our body and into our cells, now it's a simple journey from inside the cell, where they originated, to the outside of the cell. Here the exosomes encounter the cells of our immune system and are engulfed by them. End of story!

Now do you realise why it was all so confusing? Yes, viruses exist, but they don't behave remotely in the way that we have been being told they do. They are particles generated by diseased cells to play an essential role in the internal cleaning up process of those cells.

Are you saying that what doctors call "viruses" are actually exosomes? How long has science known of the existence of exosomes? Most people have not heard of them until now. I don't think medical science has related them to viruses at all. Do you think viruses and exosomes are different things?

As more and more electron microscopy images have been studied, researchers have come to realise that some of the particles seen in and around the cell membrane are moving from the inside out. This is why they have been given the name exosomes. Some scientists say these exosomes look very much like the entities that have been being called viruses. As far as research on extremely small particles is concerned this means that when examining both, they extract from exosomes and from viruses nothing more than short, single strands of genetic material (DNA or RNA) and some protein structures. Some theorise that both types of particles could well be the same thing.

Virus theory is an example of how power over an industry is able to maintain a lie and to fabricate an entire world view within society, which then shapes society itself. If you provide a group of researchers with a good laboratory and research material and tell them what they are researching are viruses, they will come and tell you what they think they've discovered about viruses. If you then do the same thing with another group of researchers in an equally good lab and tell them that what they are researching are exosomes, is this group going to know about the existence of the other group, let alone what that other group is researching? If in addition you also control the publication and dissemination of information via the media, then it's not surprising that people have no idea what is really going on. Generally, what is required is an outsider to both worlds so that an information link between the two can be created. This would allow the powers that be, the authorities, to scientifically question their own knowledge and expertise. This is common sense, but that is in short supply in recent times.

Now we have two names for the same thing, and researchers are investigating both separately. That is mind-boggling. From what you have explained, am I right to deduce that "viruses/exosomes" cannot be considered dangerous entities?

🐛 Of course. Viruses, which as we now know are generated by the cells themselves, are not dangerous. On the other hand, the appearance of those exosomes/viruses inside cells are signs that the cells are not functioning normally. In other words, they are sick. The virus did not make the cell sick. The virus is a result, the manifestation of the fact that the cell is sick.

When many cells get sick at the same time and expel those viruses, could this be a danger to nearby cells? As a consequence, could those cells also end up getting sick?

🐛 A virus is an exosome, meaning that it moves from the inside outwards. When an exosome is outside of a cell, another cell will not allow it entry. Therefore, viruses in the extracellular environment are totally harmless to surrounding cells. What we should be concerned about is the actual cause of disease in those cells. The surrounding cells receive energetic messages from their diseased neighbours, so they respond to the exosomes in a similar way in order to try and protect themselves against the specific circumstances in which all those cells are functioning at the time. They are all under the same threat. All of them, en masse, respond in the same way, so they produce the same kind of exosomes. These are expressions of the cells under the specific circumstances in which they are functioning. The circumstances are the damaging factors. Viruses are just an expression of the effect those circumstances have on those cells.

But can a virus be manipulated and thus become dangerous?

-● Viruses change all the time, naturally. We are told that they mutate. This means that, for reasons unknown to scientists, the sequences of DNA/RNA contained in those little bags are always different. Every time someone happens to look, they "discover" a new sequence and a "new" virus is born. Experts tell us that there is not just one coronavirus, but that there are many different coronaviruses, and that the reason for this is that the DNA sequence, the only defining element of a virus, is not exactly the same in one sample as in another.

The real explanation is much simpler. When a cell gets sick, what it does is to try and restore its function by doing some repair work to its structure. In the case of viruses, the cell is trying to re-establish good genetic communication within itself. What it does is to get rid of faulty or inappropriate sequences by encapsulating them to render them harmless, so that they can be expelled from the inner workings of the cell. Within the same group of cells, these inappropriate sequences will be the same. However, at a different time within the same group of cells or in a different group of cells, in a different sample of the same organism, these sequences may vary. Recalling that viruses in the external environment are never a danger, the key fact is that cells are simply throwing away their unwanted bags of rubbish.

Fear kills

The answer to your question is yes, it is possible to manipulate a virus. It is obvious that DNA/RNA sequences can be created in laboratories, but this is not a danger to living cells. Despite what some would like to believe, viruses cannot be used as biological weapons. It is true that they were tested for that purpose, but it was quickly discovered that they are completely useless for that. However, they can be used very effectively to make people sick if you can convince them they are facing an invisible deadly enemy. Fear kills, and those deaths – caused by fear, can be used to "demonstrate" a viral attack on the population. Magic tricks?

You may ask that if there is no danger to health, why people working with viruses in laboratories need such elaborate protective clothing. What is dangerous is not inert viruses but continuous contact with highly toxic chemicals in solid, liquid form or in contaminated air.

The most effective non-weapon, non-explosive warfare is not biological warfare but chemical warfare. Even the use of bacteria such as anthrax is an "amateur" way of trying to eliminate people on a large scale. When we come into contact with unusual bacteria, most people quickly adapt to them and survive. Thus, viruses are completely useless for warfare.

Chemicals, on the other hand, are highly effective. In fact, in all supposedly large-scale viral epidemics and infectious diseases, scientists have discovered, subsequently of course – that chemical poisoning was the real cause. It is also important to remember that every time something like this is published, even in the most reputable medical journals, it is quickly buried under the purported "discovery" of a new virus causing the disease. Examples include polio, mad cow disease, AIDS and now coronavirus.

You say that fear kills. That's very easy to say. But how does fear kill? Most people would say this is nothing more than a metaphor.

This has to do with the idea of "immune response" that the medical profession uses to back up its theory of immunity and resistance to disease. Medical research has, in studies specifically set up for this purpose, demonstrated that fear consistently and dramatically lowers the values obtained in immune responses. Some studies show that fear can reduce the resistance to disease by up to 80%. Most studies suggest an increased vulnerability to disease by 40-60%. Some psychology studies show that people become less resilient in dealing with stressful situations when fear consumes them.

In this regard, it is worth mentioning historical observations of smoking and serious lung disease. The greatest peak in cigarette smoking occurred during the industrial revolution in the early 20th century, whereas the largest peak in lung diseases occurred in the late 1950s and 1960s, shortly after massive advertising campaigns had been launched through billboards, radio and television, about the negative effects of tobacco smoking. Fear keeps us alive. When you are faced with a life-threatening situation it is fear that keeps you on your toes and at the peak of your capabilities. However, nature only foresees such situations lasting very short periods of time: either you escape from the threatening situation, or you succumb to it. When you survive, calm returns, you relax and carry on as if nothing has happened. The fear that is present in human beings, and that kills us, is either fear of something we cannot eliminate from our lives or fear of something we cannot perceive, an invisible enemy. The former is a battle we can't win. We put all our energy into it, but we know there is nothing we can do and we run out of energy. The second involves a continuous state of fear, because we don't know exactly when we're going to be attacked, what will happen or what we can do to protect ourselves. This is a desperate situation. On constant alert and not finding moments of true tranquillity, we run out of energy.

Everything in nature is capable of either sustaining life or taking it away. This includes water and sunlight. Everything in nature is destined to have ups and downs, powerful moments and weak moments. These include moments of stress, and the greatest feats are performed during the most intense states of stress. Nature also includes moments of rest and peace when we are regaining strength. Thus, it is the regular presence of fear and stress, in our lives that kills us. Such states are not the norm in nature.

Who are the experts advising governments? Who are these professionals appointed as medical experts in this whole coronavirus affair? Can their "expert opinions" be considered scientific?

Experts are always carefully selected. A person is appointed as an expert by his or her group of colleagues. They declare that in their opinion this person represents what they think is right. In other words, today's experts have gone through a selection process of years, the years it has taken them to gain the trust of their colleagues and to convince them that they can be trusted to say and to do the right things.

There are two types of medical experts who are advising governments: virologists and epidemiologists. Neither of them – and this is important, directly treat or care for patients. The virologists work in laboratories and epidemiologists play with statistics. The "field" doctors, such as lung specialists or intensive care doctors, have been specifically forbidden to talk on this topic. During the first few weeks, many critical and outraged comments were published expressing indignation from several high-ranking academics, as well as heads of clinical departments, such as hospitals, but these comments were immediately silenced and have never been made public again. One gets the feeling that expert advice has to be kept away from clinical information, in order not to confuse "the experts" with so much clinical experience from treating of viral infections in the population.

These experts have not been selected or appointed by governments. It is the medical profession that provides these selected experts to governments, thereby ensuring that the dissemination of information worldwide is identical and wrapped up in the same rhetoric. This makes it appear as if, despite national borders, all the world's experts are in agreement, which creates the impression that there is only one "real" version, which obviously has to be the true version.

Virologists live in a world apart, a closed world of virtual reality. They never really "see" what they are talking about – viruses – which allows assumptions to creep in among the received truth without anyone really noticing. For example, virologists still believe they do indeed isolate viruses. However, every time they have been forced to publish exactly how they have done it, which they always desperately try to avoid, the scientific community has withdrawn their articles. They always make fundamental scientific errors that allow them to believe they have isolated particular viruses, but the reality is that they have never been able to demonstrate the true origin of what they think they have found. Virologists enlighten the rest of us about viruses, their behaviour and their effects, knowledge to which only they have access. By keeping virologists away from any clinical environment and from any source of clinical information, the medical profession has at its disposal an entire army of professionals dedicated to keeping alive the story of the viruses the medical profession invented. They develop new techniques and new interference plans, always focusing on "progress". These are far from the real starting point, the basics of what a virus actually is and what it isn't, what it does and what it doesn't do. Always be on the lookout for the exceptions they find, which they present as new information, as progress in their research.

As for epidemiologists, they are statisticians who work with computer models to predict the future. The accuracy of their predictions depends entirely on how those models are designed. Whatever the desired outcome is, it is always possible to design and programme a model that provides that result. If a high value is needed, it can be arranged. If a low value is desired, that can be arranged. Like virologists, epidemiologists, have also been professionally removed from circulation, given pristine offices in exchange for specific results. These experts don't know anything about the outside world and have no way of relating what they do in their cubicles to the everyday reality in which they live.

Real science is made up of a lot of theories. It is common practice to embrace all existing theories on a subject as long as they have not yet been proven to be incorrect. True scientists may prefer a particular theory, but they will recognise that it has not been proven to be correct and they will accept that a different theory cannot be dismissed out of hand. This means, for example, that a true scientist can, on one hand tell us that he believes a particular virus is causing a specific disease in humans because it is spreading via water droplets expelled by infected people, and at the same time tell us she does not have any definitive proof that her theory is correct and that there is a possibility that it is not. A scientist will never impose her opinion on an entire population, as she herself cannot be completely sure of what she believes to be true. She is still investigating her theory.

All this leads us to the conclusion that these experts appointed by the medical profession, to the exclusion of any of their medical colleagues, are specifically chosen because they are not scientists. They are working for an employer who has given them a unique and highly visible responsibility. Their employer is in the laboratory research industry.

There is a lot of talk about "immunity" and/or "resistance" to the virus. What do these concepts mean? Are they synonymous?

In people's minds, and let's not forget that doctors are people too, immunity means "to be protected against an infectious disease". However, medical science has not been able to provide us with any evidence of what "absolute immunity" means in real terms. In other words, the medical profession has not been able to perform standard tests by which the degree of protection against disease can be determined.

Basically, three different tests are used in relation to supposed immunity, immunoglobulin tests, antibody tests and T-cell tests. The principle of all three is the same: if the results indicate a high level of activity, the message is "that you are protected". However, researchers have to continually insist that the test results do not have a direct correlation with protection, let alone immunity. It turns out that none of these tests can link high test result values to the fact that there is real protection. In a medical setting, these tests are not used to check the person's immunity, but rather to test the person's "immune response". In other words, they use the tests after a specific event such as a vaccination, or following the appearance of clinical signs of infection in order to check for the existence of a higher than usual level of activity in what they call the immune system. This is a primitive way of saying there is a "reaction". However, in order to draw real conclusions about the results of these tests in terms of "protection", this has to be seen in perspective.

It has been observed that the results of these tests return to their "normal" values quite quickly, leaving the profession totally mute when people ask "whether they are immune or not". In other words, the test results do not indicate someone's level of protection. Moreover, doctors find that, even if tests show high values, many people become infected. On the other hand some people with very low levels appear to be completely protected, even to the point that repeated attempts to inoculate their bodies with specific infectious diseases have failed. While doctors use these tests to check for what they call an immune response, they can't be sure of "disease resistance" this way.

Remember that doctors are still working from the theory that when one has been physically in contact with an infected person, one's own system must show some kind of response, either of infection or of signs the body is fighting back against the intruder. Let me present you with a scientific fact about how resistance against disease works in nature. In experiments a very specific infection was introduced into one particular tree at the centre of a forest. The scientists knew that in response to that infection, that tree would generate a very specific protein to help protect it against that disease. Once the infection had been introduced, scientists immediately measured the levels of that specific protein in the tree. As expected, they found an increased level. However, before long, they also measured high levels of that same protein in all the other trees of the same species in the surrounding area, even in those bordering the forest. The scientists were aware that there was neither physical contact between the trees nor enough time for the first artificially infected tree to become diseased. Even so, all other trees of the same species showed an immune response to an infection present *within their environment*. This demonstrates that an immune response can occur without any direct contact, providing protection against disease, even in the case of low test values. No contact is needed and high levels of "protective proteins or cells" are not required. After the initial reaction, our entire system prepares itself to recognise the danger. Unfortunately, the medical profession cannot confirm this kind of protection with any of their tests.

Is correlation the same as causation?

▶ No, it is not. That two connected things happen does not prove that one causes the other. It is too easy to use circumstantial evidence. The fact that I pay taxes to the government does not make me responsible for the arms sales the government profits from. There is, of course, a correlation between me paying taxes and the manufacturing of weapons, since that manufacturing is financed by my tax money, but my participation does not make me responsible. Similarly, the principle of "innocent until proven guilty" should be present in all scientific research. A theory remains accepted as a possibility until it is proven false. As far as infectious diseases are concerned, investors who saw profit in the system proposed by Louis Pasteur decided that there was no need for the "principle of innocence". They started to use the media, publications and rhetoric as their main weapons without any regard for the truth, thus eliminating all other possible theories.

Extending conclusions beyond the scope of an area of study became common practice.

If you manage to identify a particle that has previously been said to be responsible for a certain disease, then you have "proved" the theory! I am afraid that such a thing is absurd, from a scientific point of view and a legal point of view. First, you point a finger at something or someone, claiming that they are dangerous. Then you prove their presence at the scene of the alleged crime. Then, without further ado, you accuse them of being responsible for the crime. Yes, there is a correlation between an infection and the presence of bacteria. When bacteria are not present in diseased tissue, doctors speak of inflammation. When bacteria are present in diseased tissue they speak of an infection. This shows a clear correlation between infection and bacteria. The very definition of the term "infection" includes the presence of bacteria. However, in spite of all efforts made over two entire centuries to try and prove that bacteria are the "cause" of infections, no proof for such a statement has ever been found. Not once has science succeeded in fulfilling all the conditions required for adequately proving a cause-effect relationship between bacteria and infections. This poses a real problem in the sense that it undermines the very definition of infection. Even in many so-called "infections" there was no presence of bacteria at all. This is quite embarrassing for those who are convinced every infection is always caused by a microbe.

Okay, Mr. Expert, here you have an infection. Where is the microbe? How can I have an infection if the cause of the infection is not present? Some other type of microbe needed to appear on the scene that, for obvious reasons, could not be detected in the tests, but could be accused of causing infection. They found a candidate and they named it a "virus". It can't be seen. It can't be detected, but it is assumed that it is the cause of the infection. This creates the perfect situation for supporting the theory of infection. You have an infection. You look for the microbial culprit. You find a bacterium and say it is the cause of the infection. Or, you don't find any microbes and then assume the cause is a virus. This overlooks the fact that you have never scientifically proved a causal relationship between an infection and the involvement of a microorganism. Therefore, why would there exist a causal relationship between an infection and a virus when this is undetectable by any laboratory procedure? It is impossible to prove.

What then is the scientific evidence of infectivity that would support all the draconian measures imposed around covid19?

➤ There is no evidence! There are only theories that have been stated as facts. "It is spread through droplets we expel." "It spreads through surfaces on which it "survives" until it comes into contact with our hands." "It even spreads when there are no symptoms." "It is transmitted from animals to humans and from humans to animals." "You can also get infected through your eyes." "It can enter your body through your digestive system." "It can spread through drinking water." None of these theories have ever been proven. In fact, some, such as the surface area theory, the asymptomatic theory and the transmission from animals to humans theory have been clearly disproven. Airborne spread has only been demonstrated in cases of violent droplet expulsion by very sick people during a sneezing fit or violent coughing. This is a way of transmitting particles, true, but it is not proof that these particles are actually causing diseases.

Why do we embrace so many theories? Why, as certainly seems to be the case, as soon as someone suggests another way of transmission, has it been immediately included in the list of potential dangers?

➤ This is because they are only theories, theoretical models which, as long as no one refutes them, cannot be discarded by science. If someone were to say that you were more likely to die from COVID-19 if you were right-handed, that theory could not be discarded until someone proved it wrong. From looking at the numbers, you could make the following statements: "Black people are more prone to covid19" or "Poor people are more susceptible". If you want to use that "statistical information" before anyone has the chance to disprove the information provided, you could explain that those tendencies are due to the fact that those people have less access to adequate health care. That would, of course, be because of the shameful behaviour of the white authorities who control "proper" health systems.

To better understand the thinking behind the theories that underlie the measures taken, it is worth questioning and analysing the issue in more detail. For example, when the medical profession claims to have found evidence that the virus can be spread from animal to human, the question must be asked: "How did they come up with that evidence?" When you read how they came to find out, it goes something like this: "We grew the virus in a culture in the lab. Then we injected a high concentration of that mixed culture into animals and 65% of the animals showed signs of disease." Are these circumstances natural? Is that how it happens in life, in nature? No, that is not a scientific experiment fit to justify the conclusions they reached.

Observation is still a powerful scientific tool and we can all observe. I can observe that when 10 people in a room are exposed to whatever it is a sick person in the room is exhaling, not all of them get sick. How can that exposure be a "causal link"? We are constantly surrounded by an environment full of microbes, toxic substances and pollution, but very few people get sick. I also know that in the more sterile environments that we human beings have been creating, we are also encouraging the emergence of more dreaded microbes. The transmission theories on which they rely do not have enough evidence for proof. In fact, they are obsolete theories.

If viruses, or exosomes, are not dangerous, do not cause disease, and there is no direct transmission between people, why do you think some people are recorded as dying from COVID-19?

➤ I believe that people die when their lives have come to an end. I don't believe we have all been given the "right" to reach the average age of life. Each life ends when it is sure to come to an end, although people do feel that if a life ends as a result of an accident, it has been cut short before its time. Often when someone dies at "only" 62 their relatives want to believe that their life was cut short by illness. To me, dying from an illness should be a clear sign that life can no longer continue in the way it was going.

I know that doctors are trained in a different belief and that they want us to believe that life can be "prolonged". However, if you look carefully, you will see that it all depends on the point of view from which the analysis is made. If you believe everyone has the right to live to the age of 80 then living to the age of 62 means life has been shortened. If you look at someone at the end of their life, whether they are 62 or 80, and you notice that they have no energy or motivation left, that means that that their life has come to an end. Human beings have no power to decide how long they will live or how they can achieve a long life. We like to think we do have that power, and that is why we are going to have to prepare ourselves to learn a lot more about life and nature.

Labelling a person with a certain disease or a certain cause of death is typically human. Nature doesn't care what you call the way a life ends. It means nothing, even if one believes that life has ended as a result of infection, depression, intense sadness, starvation, poisoning, unfortunate accident or anything else. The only reality is that a life is over. Nature does not need labels. Humans need labels. Or at least, humans who need to order, separate, divide or control need labels. Livestock don't need identification tags in order to live. Humans need to brand their livestock to show who owns them. Statisticians may want to know what you're dying of but you don't need that. That's not what matters to you. For them, however, it is "vital" so that they can classify deaths, and this allows others to control or manipulate situations. A sick person has no use for a COVID-19 test result. Because there is no specific treatment for viral infections, it doesn't matter what you call a disease. A test is only useful to those who need information for separating and controlling the masses.

Why do you think more health workers have become ill than the rest of the population?

-● Remember the fear factor. Health workers are forced to go to work every day while being told that the environment in which they have to work is deadly dangerous. This goes on day after day. Health workers fear for their lives but "have" to be there. Moreover, they receive the information that that the danger is increased with increased exposure time. They are told that it is a deadly disease and the graphs "prove it". They are informed about how best to protect themselves in a deadly environment. They are told they must put on the space suits seen on television, but then at work all they have at their disposal are paper masks and plastic gloves. Propaganda infiltrates their minds for weeks and months and they end up exhausted and scared to death.

Even their own superiors, people who are supposed to know more than they do, tell them that they are not protected, but that nothing can be done for them. Do you still wonder why so many health workers have become seriously ill and why many of them have not managed to survive?

What do you think of the general recommendations by health authorities to prevent "transmission and infection"?

-€ In fact, what we have been experiencing seems to be an ideal situation for installing completely new behaviours in the population. They have been taking the opportunity to turn everything around and people simply accept it. The health authorities know for sure that it works, because for decades they've been turning established beliefs around, one by one, to see if people either comply with what they are told or if they rebel against it. First, we were told that the midday meal is the most important meal of the day, then that it's dinner. Then they switched to breakfast. No one flinched. We were given a food pyramid to tell us how to eat in a healthy way, and then they turned that pyramid upside down. Nobody has questioned that either. It seems that, in the name of progress, people are willing to accept almost anything without protest.

Now is the time to change society as a whole. What is the most worrying thing for any government? It is that people congregate. That could mean riots. If people decide things for themselves that is a nightmare because it means diversity. People seeking out what is best for them implies individuality. Having freedom of expression implies people having a variety of ideas.

What would be the ideal situation for governments? That we all do the same, think the same and believe the same things?

-€ A medical emergency. Everyone in danger. No one knowing what to do, except the government, which has the "experts" at its disposal. "Don't worry, we will rescue you, but you will have to do what we tell you or else you will not survive. As you all want to survive, you will have to trust us to take care of you. This means you will have to help us to eliminate people we will identify as being a danger to us all."

A medical emergency is the perfect situation to reverse, in one go, all the fundamental principles of our society. We all need fresh air, but no, stop, go back inside, stay indoors. When you go outdoors, wear your mask, even if it means breathing in a lot more carbon dioxide than you should (air pollution in our cities is nothing compared to breathing in your own outbreaths). We all need movement, but don't. Stop, stand still and stay at home. We all need social contact, but no, stop, it's too dangerous. Those people can potentially kill you. Everyone needs physical contact with others for their physical and mental well-being, but no, beware. Those people can potentially kill you.

There is no such thing as "social distance" or "safe distance between two people". There may be people for whom close contact is potentially a problem, but not for society at large. Keeping people apart is a common procedure in prisons. Isolation is a punishment. We know what it does to people's minds. We know that mental pain is the worst kind of torture.

Isolation causes psychological pain. It has no health benefits. On the contrary, it weakens people's spirits and capacity for determination. It turns them into dummies. It makes people docile and co-operative.

Nobody seems to care about the quality of the air we breathe. The lousy air breathed when using a mask is supposed to be for one's own "benefit". Before all this air pollution caused serious illnesses, so they told us. Not now. Now, poor air quality is "saving" lives.

Mountains of plastics no longer seem to be a problem either. We are producing more plastic than ever before, for example plastic gloves, plastic containers for gels to kill viruses, plastic face shields and plastic bags sealed to prevent contamination. This has become an essential part of our lives. Plastic no longer pollutes our environment: instead it "saves" lives.

If you really want to keep yourself healthy, you have to do the opposite of what governments are recommending. The question to ask yourself is whether you should be more afraid of the virus or the government.

What treatments are available against "viral infections" and how many lives are they saving?

➥ There is no treatment. There is no effective antiviral treatment in the medical arsenal. Doctors have been trying their best to treat the symptoms, but there is nothing available that "reduces the viral load" inside the cells and nothing to "stop the virus from multiplying". Note that I don't say anything about killing the virus because you cannot kill something that is not alive! The medical profession is focussing on "how to stop the virus from reproducing", because they believe the virus comes in from the outside, infiltrates the system and hijacks the replication system of an ordinary cell. They have been trying to find a solution to this for five decades, but the result has been a big zero. I think this should encourage rethinking the premise on which their work is based but instead they continue insisting on the same assumption and overloading scientific literature with promising stories and corrupted studies without any accountability.

Have lives been saved through their approach? No, not a single one. How can I be so sure of that? It is backed up by what government officials backed by chosen experts have said. Before they imposed lockdown and other restrictive measures they told us we needed such measures to protect the health care system. The measures were supposed to slow the spread of the disease, thus preventing everyone from getting sick at the same time and avoiding overcrowding hospitals. We were told that adopting these measures would not reduce the number of deaths or the number of people infected but that it would flatten out the curve of cases. The infection would take a few more weeks to move through the population, instead of having it all happen at once. They knew such measures would not save lives or protect anyone from the disease. They also knew that after very many weeks being locked in our isolation cells, we would be willing to settle for almost anything. They were right. Now they talk about the lives that have been saved thanks to the drastic measures and how much worse things would have been if they hadn't done it that way. Nobody seemed to protest. People seemed to be grateful for their "intelligence and foresight." It is a tall tale of invented success. Moreover, as the media, the "source of information" to which almost the entire population has given full credibility, has also remained dormant on the subject, allowing the perpetrators to walk away scot-free and in complete control of the situation.

Do you think they intended to kill a large part of the population with these measures?

-🍂 I don't think that was the main objective, but that is just my personal opinion. I don't think they cared about how many people were left at the end of all this. I think what they care about is the "class" of people they are dealing with. I think this is an exercise in power-grabbing by those already in charge of the medical system, the media and the food production system. What those groups want people to believe is nothing more and nothing less than what they say they must believe. They want total obedience. Whether a lot of people die or not is not the main issue. Those who die cease to be a concern for the powers that be. But do keep in mind that a population is needed in order to exercise power. There will be survivors, most of whom will be able to play a useful role in the new world they wish to create.

What do you recommend? What can we do as people who are becoming aware of what is going on?

-🍂 We are not all the same, not a harmoniously homogeneous group and so I can't recommend anything we all should do. I don't believe that this torrent is going to stop. I think it will continue, whatever we do. From now on the world is going to be different and I think we should be asking what the "world is going to be like". I think it would be a world of total domination, absolute control, without any individual freedom. I don't think it could be organised around restrictive laws but mainly through social control. People themselves, fearful of losing their privileges, would demand that others adhere to the rules as well. Everyone would have to "prove" they are complying with the rules in order to be able to access services and privileges, as is already happening now in some countries with the introduction of health passports. If you don't comply, you are out. In that kind of world, the crucial question would be: "To comply or not to comply?" In other words, people would have to decide whether to stay in or to get out. If you are outside, nobody would be able to help you and you would not be entitled to anything.

My sense is that all of this is an invitation for us to create a new world, a world based on different principles, totally opposite to the world we choose not to belong to. I would venture to suggest that some of the central themes for that new world should be freedom and individual respect. Everyone can fill in the details as they see fit. I see this as a radical split, a complete departure from the old society. I believe that at the moment it would be wise not to make any drastic decisions, but rather to allow our minds to consider possibilities.

The practical side of all this will be shown when we see more clearly where the world is going and who is in control. Then. each of us will have to decide whether we see ourselves living – or not, in the old way. If we cannot live in that fashion and we need to get out of it, I am sure we will find ways to do so. I recommend not trying to convince anyone who prefers to avoid what we consider to be right. Be tolerant of people who need to try things their own way. Seek cooperation where possible and allow others the freedom to live as they wish. We must allow each other the opportunity to try what we think is best. For now, let us try to keep in touch with people who do not yet seem fully convinced about all this or in full personal control of their lives. Let us not impose our ideas on anyone. Let us keep keep doors open, seeking cooperation, not differences. Let us be patient. This phase may not last that long.

As we speak Patrick, almost two years after the WHO declaration, we are still officially in a "global pandemic". How do you see the social situation at the moment? Where are we going?

➥ The old principle of "divide and rule" is the guiding principle. Keep people apart. Don't let them interact freely. Don't give them a platform where they can freely express their ideas. Isolate individuals, for example with online education. Isolate groups, for example with camps for "people considered dangerous". Control all communications. Reward "good behaviour", which can take the form of alerting the authorities to non-compliance by individuals working for the authorities in control-oriented jobs such as the police service, or in policy enforcement jobs such as social services. Restrict as much as possible, and then use very small relaxations of restrictions as rewards. Punish whole groups for the supposed "misbehaviour" of a few. Make people work very hard to gain advantages and privileges, but then remove them at the slightest infringement. If you want to get a good idea of where all this is going, watch the beginning of Roman Polanski's film *The Pianist*, about the way the Nazis managed to track down Jews in Poland at the beginning of World War II by making them wear identification bracelets.

Vaccines: a means to an end

What do you think of the vaccines they are injecting into populations?

➥ This is just another step on the road to total domination. They need the vaccination programmes to force total submission, not so much for the chip that may be in the vaccine, but for the health passport. Everything will be recorded, and the result will determine your life. Vaccination programmes are simply a means to an end. However, there is a weak point – an uncertainty, in the whole operation. This is not the fact that there will be enormous numbers of adverse effects and many deaths. That is a factor already known to the authorities. No, the key point is whether they will manage to keep the real information away from people's consciousnesses.

The real truth is about the side effects and the impossibility of providing immunity to anyone. As long as cherry-picked and modified news about negative effects of vaccines is all that reaches the public through official communication channels, the authorities will not really be questioned. However, if the testimonies become so numerous that they spread rapidly through the population and people "realise everyone else also knows people who have been negatively affected", then not only will central power collapse, but the entire Western medical system will disintegrate within a short period of time.

Some believe that they can modify our DNA and turn us into transhumans, mutant humans.

Any change in the biology of an organism is brought about by an interaction between information from the environment and the organism's reaction – individually – to that information. Therefore, the final effect within any organism is always a manifestation of the organism itself, instigated – by information from the environment. From this we can conclude that no change can take place in any organism that the organism has not created itself. Extreme environmental forces can destroy life, but alterations always occur with the consensus of the organism. Vaccines cannot therefore alter cellular DNA. However, I should add that the DNA of cells can be altered, but not through physical means such as injecting a protein structure into an organism. As all alterations are done by the organism itself, it is the individual person's state of mind that determines physical structure and function. Narratives can alter people's minds, and this, in turn, can alter their DNA. Turning people into helpless human beings, totally dependent on help from authorities, will have a profound effect on their constitutions, the design of which is contained in their DNA. Therefore, if people's behaviour changes, the energy that creates that behaviour will also change and the new energetic balance will be inscribed into the DNA.

Ultimately it is media propaganda that alters our DNA, but only if we allow it to rule our minds. In any case, using the term transhuman in relation to human beings makes no sense at all, since so far nobody has developed any technique to incorporate a piece of artificial DNA into every cell of the entire human body! Introducing the same piece of artificial DNA into 70 billion cells at a time is not something science has come close to, far from it.

That's why they are doing it "the easy way", i.e. through processes for changing minds, call it conditioning or mind programming.

Finally, I hear many reports of deaths directly caused by vaccines. Is this really happening? Don't the doctors, health workers and citizens see what is really happening?

�‣ Yes, of course it is happening. Those deaths become called new outbreaks, strains, waves or whatever you want to call them. Doctors and health workers know about it, but the authorities they work for, the authorities that pay their salaries and keep them in their status, tell them:

1. It was to be expected that some would have a bad reactions to the vaccine, so nothing out of the ordinary is happening.

2. The deaths are being caused by underlying pathologies, not the vaccine.

3. Although many vaccines have side effects, this vaccine is particularly safe. Few cases have been reported (of course, because they have only just started to happen).

Anyone in the profession who dares to speak out publicly will be severely reprimanded for spreading fake news. They are very likely to be threatened with losing their jobs and not being able to work in the healthcare world again. Silence is the price they must pay for being the system's hired guns.

The Empirical

The experimental was the first, and is the one that still retains some credit in the ordinary; because many times one sees with an herb or some other simple remedy, cures of diseases considered incurable in the other sects, or medicated situations over a long period of time without any relief. [...]

The deception of the empirical lies hidden in the confidence they have that they can cure with the same secret method all the patients of the same illness, and that the same recipe that cured Francis will also restore Anthony to health:

but at last they warn, that what served as an antidote to the former, causes harm to the latter, and that their medicines cannot be trusted in such cases to be of any profit; for the difference of climate, season, temperament, and age, is not to be relied upon as a remedy, temperament and age cause very different effects. [...]

Yesterday and Today.
El mundo engañado por los falsos medicos
Extract from the book
(The extract continues in chapter 6 and 7)

VII

THE KING OF ALL DISEASES: CANCER

There is a disease that everyone is afraid of. Western medicine has – allegedly – been trying to find a cure for decades, raising tons of money for research. I say "allegedly" because it seems that, having invested so much time and so much money in research, very little has been achieved, There is still no "cure" and many people are still dying of cancer, often after long, expensive and painful chemotherapy treatments. Please speak about cancer.

➤ Cancer is a disease that is spreading through modern society like wildfire. We are encouraged to financially support all efforts to combat the horrors that accompany it, and yet, despite the best efforts made by "so called experts" – cancer doctors, oncologists and researchers – over the last forty years, the general consensus has been that we are losing the battle against cancer. In fact, this cry is echoed across all fields of serious disease. Although it has been repeatedly promised, there is still no cure for multiple sclerosis, diabetes, rheumatoid arthritis, Parkinson's disease, heart attacks, asthma and other serious conditions. I am not talking about "containing the disease" or "monitoring it". I am talking about <u>curing it.</u> Unfortunately, the population has ended up even accepting terrible words from the medical authorities about there being no cure.

Annual statistics show that the incidence of cancer is increasing, not diminishing, despite the many celebrated medical advances of recent decades. The explanation given for the obvious fact that there is more cancer now than ever before is that "they are much better at detecting it now". In other words, the medical profession's position is that there is no more cancer than before but simply that detection is better. However, when the rest of us use this same argument to justify the apparent current increase in infectious diseases, then this argument is vehemently rejected by those same authorities. They decide when the argument is valid and when it is not.

In reality, the only data that would prove they are "getting it right" would be cancer survival statistics. These statistics show the five-year survival rate of cancer patients. They seem to show that more and more people are surviving cancer, year on year. However, "survival", in clinical terms, indicates that the person lives for at least five years from the day they were diagnosed. Dying one day after five years is considered a success, and the case is recorded as a cancer survivor. You may find this hard to believe, but suffering from cancer for twenty years is recorded as having survived cancer four times! Thus, the cancer survival numbers are greatly amplified and are not a measure for curing cancer.

Here is an interesting question: "Which procedure is most emphasised in the fight against cancer?" What is the most powerful "weapon" they have for achieving "fantastic" survival figures? The answer is early detection. Why? Because early detection increases the survival rate enormously. It means that you are much more likely to be alive five years after the date of diagnosis. This leads directly to statistics with supposedly "positive" results, which is what the medical authorities want to see.

It always takes time for a cancer to remove the life from our system because our organism resists the disease with all its might. The innate healing power of an organism will cling to life in any way possible, until the last breath. Even if you do nothing specific to "fight" cancer, your body will always work in your favour, in favour of living. This means any cancer is going to need quite a long time to kill you, a great deal of time from its inception to the final collapse of your system. If we apply the five-year rule, the sooner the cancer is discovered, the more time you have before your life is over, and consequently the more chance you have of "surviving". This makes for great statistic but it is bad news for you. Your suffering is going to be extended as you will now start to suffer from a much earlier time. Once diagnosed, you will never again live your life without stress. It is likely that your life will be completely altered as a result of the treatments and all their effects.

At the time of diagnosis, most people have no or very mild symptoms. They do not suffer. Suffering begins as soon as treatment is started. Let us remember that cancer is not just a disease of modern times. It has always existed as a disease. In the old days, most of the time doctors didn't know someone had cancer until after they had died. It is important to know that most people die with cancer, not of cancer. Doctors didn't know because their patients didn't complain. For example, women with breast cancer. Most of them continued working on their farms and applying poultices to their open wounds. No doctor was needed for that. The accepted attitude was that there was nothing that could be done, which, in modern times, has been proven to be largely correct. However, everything began to change when doctors started to have more influence in people's lives, telling them that they had to tell the doctor immediately, at the slightest symptom, always "suspecting" cancer. The medical profession began intervening much earlier, and that is when suffering began on a global scale. The more aggressive the treatment, the more extreme the suffering. The focus of life shifted away from nature, from real life, and shifted to illness and death. Cancer has always existed, but few people died from it. Most continued to live with it. From the moment the medical profession stepped in, more people died from cancer to the point where a diagnosis of cancer became a death sentence.

In almost a century and a half of specific medical treatments for cancer, nothing has changed, except that now more people do die of cancer or, to be more precise, of cancer treatments. We are told of the fantastic advances in the fight against cancer, and yet neither the protocols nor the results seem to improve patients' lives. Aside from the – manipulated – survival statistics that I mentioned earlier, cancer rates and all cancer related problem rates are increasing year by year. This is despite annual increases in resources and constant claims of breakthroughs in the treatment of specific cancers. Unfortunately, none of these claims have ever been substantiated. It is all propaganda.

The cruel reality is that we have a serious treatment problem. Their principles have not changed since the first treatments that were used against cancer. During World War II, several researchers and oncologists declared that there was no evidence that the radio-therapy and chemotherapy, which had been in use for the previous sixty years, had produced any change in outcomes. However, they did say that these treatments worsened quality of life. Eighty years later we are still doing the same things and talking in the same manner. We have made torture more sophisticated, but there has been no "breakthrough" whatsoever. Nor will there be any if the medical profession continues to use the same strategies. The "breakthrough" only applies to purely technical aspects that have nothing to do with real progress in terms of fundamental understanding. The strategy always remains the same: cut, burn and poison. However, a real "breakthrough" could very well be produced by simply looking at the disease from a different perspective.

What cancer might be

What is cancer when viewed from a different perspective?

First, let us determine what the medical profession calls "cancer". Cancer is the name of a disease and all symptoms that accompany it, caused by the existence and development of a tumour. This forms from neoplasm, the "abnormal and excessive growth of tissue that is not coordinated with the growth of the surrounding normal tissue. This abnormal growth usually forms a mass called a tumour." It is an overgrowth, uncoordinated in its functions with respect to those of the surrounding normal tissue. It grows even after the initial trigger has been removed. In other words, once the process has begun, it is irreversible. There is a suspicion of some kind of a trigger, something that sets the entire process in motion. What might that trigger be?

It has been estimated that up to 80% of human cancers are related to chemical and environmental factors. There is often a long latency period between exposure to a particular carcinogenic chemical and the development of the corresponding neoplasm, which makes it impossible, most of the time, to prove a connection between a trigger and the cancer, something the tobacco industry has always rightly argued. No real proof can ever be delivered. Hundreds of chemicals – such as additives or preservatives, used in industry, in agriculture, in the home, and in food items – are labelled as carcinogenic.

The use of radiotherapy has led to an increased incidence of acute leukaemia. This in a much shorter interval of time than in the case of the chemical links mentioned above. It has not yet been possible to determine with certainty what a safe and acceptable dose of radiation would be. It has also been shown that, in addition to an increased risk of leukaemia, patients treated with radiotherapy are at a significantly increased risk of developing thyroid carcinoma. In cases of women undergoing repeated chest X-ray, including in mammography screening programmes, or fluoroscopy examinations, an increased incidence of breast cancer has been demonstrated, even at very low radiation doses. Prenatal exposure to synthetic oestrogens has been associated with vaginal and cervical adenocarcinomas, much later in the life. Postnatal oestrogen exposure for contraception or during menopause has resulted in an increased risk of endometrial and cervical carcinoma. Oestrogens, prescribed as birth control pills, also cause liver adenomas and cancer. All cytotoxic drugs – used in chemotherapy – are known to cause cancer. Immunosuppressive drugs used in transplants, cancer treatment protocols and autoimmune diseases such as rheumatoid arthritis, cause various skin and intestinal cancers.

However, if up to 80% of all cancers are related to chemical and environmental factors, why is the profession trying to focus our minds on genetics as the origin of cancer, when biologists, in the last ten years, have concluded that genes are responsible for only a small group of diseases? The combination of genetics as a cause, and cancer as a consequence, is extremely rare, if not non-existent! So the latest trick has been to link cancer to a viral infection, for example linking cervical cancer to human papillomavirus, and so we have gone from blaming chemicals to blaming genes to blaming viruses. Now they are creating a whole new encyclopaedia of possible causes of cancer processes, using the link to viruses – those barely detectable particles that we know nothing about.

In the 1960s, scientists suggested that at any point in our adult lives there could be neoplastic cells present somewhere in our body, and that every person could develop at least one tumour in his or her lifetime. Almost all of those heal up spontaneously. Twenty years ago, their suggestion became that, over the course of a lifetime, it was very likely for humans to develop five tumours! From one to five, we are making progress. The immune status of the host is invariably named as a major factor in the development of all cancers. In other words, if the person is healthy and strong, neoplastic development has little chance of taking hold. This means that having diseased cells in our body is part of the normal cycle of our life and that no treatment is necessary.

What, in general terms, weakens a person's immune system and makes them more vulnerable to disease? Might, toxins, stress, self-doubt, lack of sunshine, lack of vitamins and minerals, vaccinations, immunosuppressive drugs, recurrent illnesses and infections be involved?

This society encourages us to increase our stress levels, resulting in fear, anger, doubt and consequent actions related to those feelings. There is no longer as much respect for others and, as a result, people have very little respect for themselves. Lack of self-esteem means having less resilience. And these mental factors seem to be much more important than any physical influences.

A new cancer story

Starting from the premise that everything is energy, a tumour is also just an expression of that energy. It is an integral part of the person who presents the symptoms. The person has grown the tumour as part of the expression of what life is like for them.

What might that expression mean? What is it telling us?

-❧ A tumour is a cluster of abnormal cells that manifests itself as hardened tissues. In many cases a tumour can be removed or isolated from the surrounding tissue as a hard, solid lump. Some normal tissue has lost flexibility and softness, solidifying and becoming much denser. The person has been stiff, with little mobility or fluidity in those specific tissues. Remember that long term, the physical expression of a change in the consistency of a tissue is related to a state of functioning that the person has consistently maintained – for a long time. The tissue where the tumour occurs is related to an aspect of life in which they have become too rigid to continue to live. We will return to that.

On a physical level, reduced flow means that everything slows down as it passes through those tissues. Water flows more slowly, blood circulation slows down and nerve signals will decrease in intensity and frequency. As a direct result, all cellular activity will be reduced. Cells will have to be patient while waiting for nutrients and instructions. In addition, because they have less flexibility in their actions, not only will the functionality of the tissues, their speed of action and their ability to react be reduced, but each action will also leave residue. Under normal circumstances this waste would simply be "swept away" by the powerful flow through the tissues. If this flow is no longer happening waste will accumulate in the tissue.

After some time this will begin to seriously threaten the normal functioning of the cells. They will now have an additional problem as well as lack of nutrients. What can you do when the rubbish truck only shows up once in a while, not frequently enough to remove the growing mountain of waste? Instead of allowing waste products to be scattered all around, taking up all the tissue, we can try to put it all in one place. This is like creating a landfill, a place in the middle where all the waste can be dumped. As the weight and volume of waste increases over time, it will become more compacted, solidified and hardened, resulting in a tumour.

Cancer is a toxic process of asphyxiation through overloading tissue with waste. It is a process, not a condition! A condition implies something static, but cancer, like life itself, is a process. It is something changeable that can keep solidifying more and more, or, on the other hand, could start to resolve itself. The cancerous process can go either way, deteriorating or healing. What is very clear is that by adding more and more toxic material to the system, we will not lighten the burden of the cancer.

Pieces of rubbish may fall off and drift away, floating in the water and blood that passes through the tumour. Most of these waste products, now in compact forms that look like abnormal cells, will be picked up by the lymph nodes that filter the water circulating in the area. Lymph nodes are local centres designed to remove waste from the water flowing between the cells. These lymph nodes are part of our cleansing system. They prevent the debris, identified by doctors as "cancer cells", from entering the bloodstream. They capture waste and break it down. Lymph nodes are essential for clearing "dirt" accumulated at a tumour site. If you have a tumour, you desperately need each and every one of your lymph nodes in order to solve the problem!

This is how nature works. Our "defences" are working and doing an excellent job. Now I am going to tell you how the medical profession acts in this situation. When doctors find waste products in the lymph nodes of their patients' bodies they panic. They are convinced that tumours, which they consider to be the enemies and the culprits of the disease, are trying to "escape", to spread and metastasise to different parts of the body. A doctor, determined to stop the spread at any cost, removes the lymph nodes, thus unwittingly eliminating the first line of defence. Once that line of defence has been eliminated, there is nothing left to control and prevent the waste products from flowing to other areas and clogging up more and more tissue. The waste has free entry to the entire body. Opening the doors of the lymphatic circulation in this way will not create secondary tumours, but it will increase the waste load throughout the body and hinder the functioning of the entire system.

If the problem of accumulated waste is contained in a particular place, at least the rest of the system can continue to function more or less normally. This is what we do in towns and cities. If there is an excess of rubbish, we accumulate it in one place and isolate it from the living population.

Cancer cell migration

When the resistance of an organism is low, it seems logical that rapid proliferation of out-of-control cells may occur. Neoplasms, understood as abnormal cell growth, will develop into tumours, balls or nodules of hardened cells. These in turn will develop into cancer, the disease process that includes all signs and symptoms related to cancer. The medical profession then assumes that some cells can detach themselves from a tumour and wander around the body until they can camp out somewhere else to start a new colony.

What causes the medical profession to determine that a second tumour, called a "secondary" or "metastatic" tumour, is not a different tumour but has its origin in the original tumour, the "primary" tumour?

Because the cancer cells of the new tumour look somewhat like those of the original tumour, they conclude that it is not a new tumour. The original tumour must have taken a journey through the body and started a new community elsewhere.

Let's imagine for a moment that some cells get fed up with living in their close-knit community. Suppose those cells decide to pack up their things, say goodbye to their friends and family and set off on a journey. How? Through lymphatic and blood circulation. They don't ask themselves many questions but just enjoy the journey. The cells travel floating in the bloodstream. How do they decide where to settle to start a new life? As there may be nothing in particular that attracts them to any particular place, we have to assume they drop out of circulation because they get stuck somewhere. We already know that certain kinds of cancers establish secondary enclaves in specific organs. If we assume cells "get stuck" in the tissue where the secondary tumours appear one might wonder why. It would be logical for cells to get stuck where the blood vessels are smallest, not where they are larger. The smallest vessels are the capillaries, through which the blood delivers oxygen to individual cells, and in which the arterial circulation becomes the venous circulation. By far the largest number of capillaries are found in the skin and digestive system. There are hardly any in bone tissue. If we compare the statistics of the occurrence of secondary tumours in various tissues, the liver, bones, and lungs are prominent sites. Perhaps cells do not travel.

Why would cancer cells want to migrate when no other cell in the body ever does that?

This does seem unlikely when they are cells that are not functioning properly. Questions about why and how cancer cells migrate haven't been answered. I would like to know how it was determined that this happens. Cancer cell migration doesn't seem to answer the question of why a secondary lung cancer could come from a breast cancer that was surgically removed a few years earlier? None of these questions have been answered.

Why is the microbiology of a secondary cancer very similar to that of the primary?

It is "very similar" but not exactly the same! Similar does not mean identical. In order for this to happen, our immune system, said to exist to protect us and fight for our lives, has to ignore these "travelling cells" and not react at all. So, apparently, in this case, our immune system (let's assume for now that it exists) stops protecting us. So far, the proponents of the "travelling cells" theory have never given an explanation for the non-reaction of such a vital part of a human being. Moreover, if such a migration of cells were possible, it would make the process of "choosing" the new settlement, of where to start the new tumour colony, a random event. Starting a new colony could, in principle, happen anywhere, and, statistically, we should find an even distribution throughout the body. However, reality tells us that this is not the case. The medical profession itself informs us that it is very predictable where the primary tumour will metastasise if it does.

- Breast cancer tends to spread to the bones, liver, lungs, chest wall and brain.
- Lung cancer tends to spread to the brain, bones, liver and adrenal glands.
- Prostate cancer tends to spread to the bones.
- Colon and rectal cancers tend to spread to the liver and lungs.

So, if it's not random, there must be a link between the various tissues that have such similar tumours. If it is not random, where is the proof that the cells that are shed from the original tumour are still alive, are able to travel and have the power to start a new colony of their own? And I repeat, where is our natural defence system in this whole process?

Are you saying cancer cells don't migrate?

�'❥ Remember that everything is energy. A cancer is a solidification of accumulated energy in the individual. Everything happening in any in any given tissue in the body is related to the type of energy that has been altered. The same mechanism is valid for secondary tumours. They are also solidifications in specific parts of our human energy field. Therefore, the secondary tumour arises directly at the place where we find it without it coming from anywhere else. There is no migration through the blood circulation. There are no travelling cells. Each tumour appears directly at the site where it is found.

Why do certain cancers "spread" to specific tissues and not to others?

�'❥ It seems as if tissues that favour the appearance of particular cancers somehow have something in common. As discussed earlier, there are seven types of tissues. All of them combine in various ways to create the seven systems of the body. In all seven systems we find the same seven energies, present in different amounts and in different combinations in each system. When we have a disturbance in a specific layer of energy, it effects all the systems of the body. Where the effect is going to be most noticeable is where more of that type of energy is present. It will be less noticeable in the other tissues. This easily explains why certain tumours, accumulations of specific cell types in a specific system, seem to spread to other systems of the body in which those cell types have similar functions. As long as the problem or pressure on that specific layer of energy remains, there is the possibility that other tissues containing less of the same energy will also begin to malfunction, and they will do so in a similar way as at the original site, since the expression of the malfunction is the expression of that type of energy.

Let's illustrate this with the energy scheme I explained earlier, in chapter 4. When, for example, energy 2 undergoes chronic pressure, it changes to a state of contraction.

What then happens to the physical manifestation of it?

1	lymphatic system	mostly 1 and 3	little of 5 and 7
4	circulation system	mostly 4 and 6	little of 5 and 7
6	feeding system	mostly 6 and 4	little of 3 and 7
2	mobility system	mostly 2 and 5 (or 6)	little of 1 and 3
5	communication system	mostly 5 and 7	little of 1 and 3
7	nervous system	mostly 7 and 5	little of 1 and 3
3	glandular system	mostly 3 and 1	little of 5 and 7

Here we see the sub-frequencies that make up each of the seven energies or frequencies.

1 Divides according to the code 1-3-4-6-2-5-7

2 Divides according to code 2-5-6-7-4-1-3 (code 2D), four possibilities.

3 Divides according to code 3-1-4-4-6-2-5-7

4 Divides according to code 4-6-1-2-3-5-5-7

5 Divides according to code 5-7-2-6-4-1-3

6 Divides according to code 6-4-2-1-5-7-3 (code 6B) two possibilities.

7 Divides according to code 7-5-2-2-6-4-1-3

Frequency 2 controls mobility, movement. It manifests itself as fat, the energy reserve that fuels all bodily activity. It also controls the locomotive system, including the muscles, joints and bones. The part of the motor system that is fully representative of frequency 2 is the pelvic area and hips. Problems with hip mobility, which lead doctors to perform hip replacement operations, are the result of a contraction (yin motion) of frequency 2.

When the primary tumour is due to a contraction of frequency 2, we will find possible secondary tumours in the regions that are relatively high in frequency 2. In the creation coding system, the composition of all the other energy layers, you can identify those that contain a high percentage of frequency 2. In frequencies 7, 6, and 5, frequency 2 reaches up to the third level. This means that the rate of occurrence of secondary tumours in the nervous system, lungs, intestines and in sensory system is not very high, but if there is going to be metastasis, it will be in those areas.

With what we now know, we can describe a tumour as the condensation of a specific energy manifested in a specific place in the body. It is a normal manifestation in the tissue, which then, as a result of the circumstances and the way someone perceives them, densifies. Therefore, cancer is always the expression of a disease of contraction. It is always the end of a long road with various signs and clues that the person has been courageously ignoring. Too much pressure in life, specifically on the energy associated with the tissue in which the tumour develops, is what can trigger the cancerous process, from neoplasm to tumour to cancer.

Knowing this, the solution, the complete cure for cancer, is to remove the intense pressure on that area of life. Because by the time of diagnosis someone has already travelled a long way to get to the stage of cancer, I would suggest not waiting too long before taking decisive action. not dispersing attention in other directions, whether or not the tumour is growing or "spreading". That is the time to make drastic decisions about the way you are living, and I recommend making major changes to your life.

The good news is that you can actually survive cancer if you are able to change the way you live, not continuing with what created the cancer in the first place. The way your tissues function is a direct result of the interplay between your outer world and your inner world. We have seen that this interaction depends, to a large extent, on the information you allow into your cells. The way you have lived, your attitudes towards certain aspects of your life, your patterns of reaction to certain circumstances, have all converged to the point at which your system is no longer able to withstand the pressure.

You need to take a good look at yourself.

You may be able to identify clearly what kind of pressure has caused the cancer in your body, or you may not. If you can, there is only one solution: eliminate it immediately. For whatever reason, you have been putting up with that pressure, but now you know that if you continue to do so, it will be the end of your life. This, as a conscious choice, is perfectly acceptable. It will allow you to end your life in peace, without too much struggle. If, on the other hand, you really don't have any idea what might have caused the cancer, then it is very likely you haven't been watching yourself very closely or it may be an accumulation of several circumstances.

I would advise you to change all the fundamental structures of your life if you want to carry on living. I am basically talking about relationships, working conditions, family life, where you live and how you live. You have two viable options and you should use both. Change your environment as drastically as you can and change your attitude as drastically as you can. You can learn to react differently to incoming information, but you also need to make sure that the incoming information is not the same as it has been.

Healing involves permanent change. There is no healing without drastic change. Not an apparent change, a quick coat of paint or a botched repair with four nails and a hammer. It has to be change to the structure of your life, the way you have been living up to that moment. The foundations on which you have built your life can no longer support you. To live is to work. Manifesting life is the only truth. If you have made changes but your cancerous process does not reverse, it means you have not been able to make the necessary changes, the ones at the heart of the problem. You don't need to take any tests. No other person can tell you whether you are improving your life, enriching it or not. You need to look at your life and learn to know it, feel it and evaluate its quality. You should not follow expert opinions or advice from books or any other source. Your heart is crying out for you to listen to it and to follow it. Trust the truth. The truth is in the manifestation of your own life.

It's hard to make a drastic change in life. Honestly, I don't think I've seen anyone do it. Do you really know of people who have cured their cancer this way? Do you think many people can do it?

�‣ You are right. It is difficult, but we only experience it as difficult because we're not used to making drastic changes. What we know, what we are used to, is easier for us. Our society doesn't care. It doesn't want us to make the drastic changes each individual needs because then we would be allowing each individual to do what they think is best for them. That would destroy the whole economics of the health system in a few months. We are not, therefore, accustomed to putting ourselves first, nor do we know how to develop ourselves as human beings. On the contrary, we are constantly reminded that we must abide by the rules, adapt our behaviour and live our lives as others think we should. Furthermore, we are told that this is out of respect and consideration for our fellow human beings. In other words, you must respect everyone except yourself!

In fact, many people have succeeded in surviving. The first cancer survival stories were told by people who had completely abandoned their old life. "If I'm going to die anyway then I don't want to end up living like this. I want to experience a different style of life!" It could be said that they survived "by chance", but their experiences have shown us the way. Decades later we can turn that into a basic law of nature. Cancer only appears when you do nothing to avoid or to stop chronic stress in your life.

In nature, animals don't get cancer. Only domestic animals get cancer, probably because they are cared for by humans. This small difference already tells us a lot.

You talk about the toxic origin of cancer. You say it has been estimated that up to 80% of human cancers are related to chemical and environmental factors. But then you talk about the pressure from the environment and you also say that the tumour is related to the aspect of life where they have become too rigid to go on living. How does one relate to the other? As I understand it, one thing is radiation or chemical toxicity or toxicity, and pressure from our outside world is another.

That perception corresponds to a physical view of the world, whereas life and nature are energy. A toxic substance is anything that is a burden to an individual in his or her life at that time. For example, alcohol is a toxic substance that makes some people sick but not others. It depends on the individual and his or her circumstances. Those circumstances are the pressures under which people live. For each person the pressures are different and, furthermore, they change throughout our lives. They do not remain stable. At some point in our lives we may have a toxic reaction to a substance, one that we have never had before and will never have again. For some people, water can be toxic. I have known people for whom air had become a toxic substance. In other words, the definition of a toxic substance also needs to change if we focus only on the individual, because the specific "toxic effect" manifests itself at a specific place in that person's physical structure. We must take into account that every part of the body is a manifestation of a specific energy. If any one of those energies becomes unbalanced, that person will become intolerant or allergic to specific substances, and when he or she shows signs of that toxicity, they will manifest in those specific areas of their body.

Here are a few more notes about the medical profession with respect to the fact that toxic substances cannot be defined by themselves. If you buy heroin on a street corner it is a toxic substance that can potentially kill you. However, if the doctor prescribes you morphine, which is pretty much the same thing – then it becomes a substance that has the potential to save your life. Artificial sweeteners occupy a prominent place in the pyramid of toxic products, but when they are used in soft drinks or cooking, the medical profession claims them as "healthy". Radioactive material is highly toxic, and people who potentially come into contact with it are carefully screened. Yet, when it is used as a "treatment", radiotherapy is seen as healthy. When some of the radiation escapes into the environment by accident we may be told that there is no danger to the population, and so on and so forth.

Are you being sarcastic about the medical profession?

There is no need for irony or sarcasm on my part: the irony is in the facts. The medical profession takes all this very seriously. They believe in what they say and do. Doctors have not been trained to think, only to believe. When we put facts together like this it always brings out the folly of their professional reasoning.

I assume you have heard of Dr. Ryke G. Hamer. His explanation of cancer is different from yours. I value the German New Medicine highly. Hamer speaks of a DHS19 – initial shock – and explains the biological programmes that lead to tumours, cancers and other diseases. Is his view compatible with yours?

Yes, it is. I will give you a more detailed explanation of why a shock, or a DHS, as Hamer would call it, results in cancer in one person and not in another. A shock is something that happens to a person. It is an incoming signal from the outside world. Here is the key point. When the shock occurs, there are two possibilities. The person allows the signal to enter their energy field and to disturb their personal energy balance, or they do not allow it. If the signal is not allowed to enter, that person will live through the traumatic event with no lasting effects. If the input is allowed, there are two possibilities. They may be able to make a major readjustment in their life to minimise the effects, or he or they may not be able to do so. Adjustment consists of altering previous reaction patterns so that their system, if it still has enough energy left, can heal. By making the appropriate adjustment, they will be able to move to a different balance and heal. If they don't make that important adjustment, the only option left to the system will be to continue to struggle to maintain an "old equilibrium" that has become impossible to maintain. This is nothing more or less than dying a slow death, spending one's last sparks of energy fighting against the reality of one's life. After a traumatic event it is never the same as before.

Taking this a step further, I can see that the traumatic event was not an accident but rather a desperate attempt by the system to prevent someone from continuing to live their life as they had been doing. If someone is still unwilling to listen, then there is not much more the system can do except to fight their stubbornness and tenacity.

In this last paragraph, I take it that when you say that "the traumatic event was not an accident" you mean that "the cancer was not an accident"? A traumatic event is not supposed to be avoidable, is it? We can't prevent things from happening.

-❧ I mean exactly what I said. The traumatic event was not an accident. And yes, I mean an accident such as someone breaking a leg, getting hit by a car or cutting off a finger. These things don't happen randomly, as most people believe. It happens because our mind is not truly present in that place and in that moment. Those things mainly happen because we are too distracted. It may be momentary, but most of the time it's things that have been on our minds for a long time, things we are not willing to let go off. Personal accidents can definitely be avoided. The only distinction to be made is between a personal accident and one that happens to a group of people. In a group, your personal involvement is much smaller and perhaps not enough to avoid the accident. One thing is for sure: luck has nothing to do with it.

It is neither bad luck nor good luck.

I am currently living through the cancer dying process of a person close to me. I am observing many character changes. A very kind, calm, diplomatic person, always helping others, has become unfriendly, impatient, very direct and too honest. I would say that he is a different person. Do you think this could be due to toxicity from the drugs he has been given? Or do you think that perhaps his brain has decided to reduce pressure from his family environment as a self-healing mechanism, the kind of pressure you talk about?

Very often there are marked personality changes in people who are at the end of their lives. This happens because they are forced to readjust and bring their life into line with what it should be. Some people, who have lived too quietly, who have been too charming and who have been too attentive to the needs of others, get the opportunity to turn inward. They focus on their own needs and develop a tendency to get angry and to behave aggressively towards their environment. We could say that, finally, they are rectifying what they had not done in their lives, i.e. spoken up for themselves and said exactly what they were thinking. Others, on the other hand, are at peace with their environments and their situations. Even though they may have been difficult to deal with or to live with, for example people who have always said what they thought, who have been stubborn, they may now be calm and at ease with life and their environment. Everything is always fine for this type of person. So, to answer your question, there is no direct effect of "toxicity" on this change of character. It is a manifestation of the person's system, which readjusts itself before the retraction of their energy field takes place.

What do you mean by this? Would you put it another way please?

If you are at ease with your surroundings, even if your environment is very turbulent and disturbing, it means that those external events are, of course, still present in your energetic field and influences it. However, your mind does not concentrate on those changes. It is not afraid of being influenced by them, and so your own energy field somehow "absorbs" the disturbing signals, bringing any possible distortion of the energy field back into its personal balance. Then there will be no physical manifestation caused by the disturbances in the external field.

When you talk about the toxicity of the body, you say that the symptoms of toxicity are going to manifest in specific areas of the body. I think this is an interesting "Pandora's box" that we need to open up. We are entering the field of intolerances and allergies, aren't we? Nowadays it is rare to find people, particularly children, who do not have an intolerance or allergy to some substance such as a food like nuts or eggs, dust, or medicines. What can you tell us about this? What can we do if we have an allergy?

Intolerance and allergy are two separate things for the medical profession. Anyone can "diagnose" an intolerance and, as you know, certain things or situations can be intolerable for us. However, an allergy diagnosis is made in a laboratory. Certain proteins in the blood may be detected. When there is a high level of specific proteins combined with a clinical picture of intolerance a diagnosis of allergy is made. In reality however, there is no difference. These intolerances are manifestations that may occur any time in life for no apparent reason. That is something the medical profession refuses to look at all. They are only interested when there is an external cause so obvious that no one can deny the evidence any longer. That reason, as you may have guessed, is toxicity. We accumulate toxicity when our system no longer knows what to do with all the waste we are generating. When someone's body is choking on a specific waste product, it's desperately important to stop it from entering the body. The body tries to avoid waste at all costs, sending warning signals that can even modify our behaviour. The system lets us know that we cannot tolerate a substance any longer. It has been able to so far, but not anymore.

Allergies and intolerances can be completely cured, disappearing completely after a strict period of cleansing. When you start to realise and discover what it is that really – energetically – makes you overreact, that's when you can change your life accordingly. Then you will never have that reaction to that substance again.

I think it's such an interesting and hot topic that perhaps deserves a separate chapter. do you agree?

🖤 Absolutely yes. You've convinced me.

The Methodists

The second sect was that of the Methodists, who believed that they could become accomplished in the Medical Faculty with very little work, and boasted that they could teach anyone in six months the entire Art of Medicine.

It was enough for them to know certain common principles and some universal knowledge, but they did not pay attention to the knowledge of the singular and the causes of ailments.

The Empirics believed that the causes could never be known, and the Methodists judged them to be fruitless; for which reason the former are worthy of pity, for confessing the weakness of their own understanding; and the latter are worthy of the same punishment, for despising as useless the investigation of causes.

Yesterday and Today.
El mundo engañado por los falsos medicos

Extract from the book
(The extract continues in chapter 9)

VIII

ALLERGIES

We live in a society of allergy sufferers and people with numerous intolerances. Nowadays it is difficult to find someone who is not allergic or intolerant to something. Restaurant menus are clear example of this with gluten-free, lactose-free, nut-free, and egg-free dishes.

🐦 Controversies over reactions to foods, and to many other substances, have been inextricably bound up with disputes over terminology. A Viennese paediatrician, Baron Clemens Von Pirquet, first used the term "allergy" in 1906, to mean altered sensitivity. This basically means any idiosyncratic response of the system to the environment. By 1925, as laboratory tests became considered to have more value than clinical observations, most of those working in the field of allergy decided to limit the definition. Only reactions in which the immune system was demonstrably altered were classified as allergic reactions. Hence the differentiation between food allergy and food intolerance. Allergy has therefore become a rather narrow science. If a patient does not provide a positive response to a scratch test (a small amount of food scratched into the skin) or a distinct antibody is not found in the blood or intestinal lining in responds to exposure to a particular food then in the minds of immunologists a food allergy cannot be the problem.

Yet, in many instances, for example coeliac disease, where no obvious conventional allergy is present, removal of an offending food does result in great improvement. This suggests that the disease is linked to the food item through some kind of immunological response, even though it cannot be demonstrated to be a "classical" allergy.

The clinical ecologist calls this a food allergy as well, often to the sound of derision from professors of immunology. Perhaps *food sensitivity* or *food intolerance* would be more sensible terminology, as neither the immunologist nor the clinical ecologist need take offence. I feel much of the debate surrounding the "allergy" issue has its roots in semantics and concepts that surround the word itself. Different specialists like to lay ownership on the term. It means different things to different people.

From a practical point of view, it is quite obvious that an allergic reaction and over-sensitivity are essentially the same thing in expression and in individual experience. Doctors diagnose allergic reactions all the time without doing extensive allergy tests, especially as a lot of these reactions occur occasionally or express themselves in different ways and are quickly dismissed as the patient gets better without any particular long-term help. We find other proof that the two are very closely related, if not exactly the same, in experimental evidence of great improvement in health from the moment contact with the offending item is totally avoided. Whatever the intricate bodily mechanism, we can categorically state that there is a direct link between contact with the substance and expression of malfunctioning in the immune system or, to be more precise, in the entire system. It is very likely that there are several possible reaction pathways for the body, but the essential point here is the direct relationship between the substance and the malfunction.

We are talking about a learned immune system response to environmental agents that are not intrinsically harmful but that, for whatever reason, the system has become very afraid of. If these "trigger-agents" are essentially innocent particles or items, how can we justify blaming the allergic reaction on the trigger?

"Why does a substance trigger an allergic reaction in one individual and not in another? Why does it do so today if it didn't in the past?"

-❧ The great majority of research into allergies has been done with respect to two aspects of the problem. On the one hand we want to know what causes allergies. This has been translated into identifying the specific trigger of an allergy. Secondly, in order to understand allergies, scientists have spent many years deciphering cellular "allergic" reactions in an effort to understand how they work and what causes them. Let's put thought into these two approaches.

It is s very interesting finding out how cells react and what chemicals are produced during an allergic reaction. However, one does not need to know what happens in the engine in order to be able to drive or make the best use of a car. Most information gained about allergic reactions is of the order of what happens and how it happens once the body's defence system makes contact with the allergen. It does not answer the question of *why* the body does what it does when most of the time, in other people in the same circumstances, it reacts totally differently. One claim we hear is that all the research is leading towards better understanding of the genetics behind the allergic disorders. Bearing in mind that allergies in adults usually develop later in life, it is difficult to "blame" them on faulty genes. Then the question of why genes would "become faulty at that stage in life" arises. The other problem this approach to allergies has caused is that it takes the focus away from disease patterns to concentrate solely on immune reactions, resulting in narrow definitions of allergy and big arguments about semantics.

Can we truly say that the trigger for the allergy is the cause of the allergy? It is certainly the cause of the allergic reaction, but is it the real cause of the allergy? Can the trigger be blamed for what happens? Can the gun be blamed for the killing? The fact that almost all identified allergy-triggers cause no such overreaction in the great majority of people, throws the idea of the trigger being the cause into serious doubt. Equally, we have to accept that one can become allergic to almost anything, which means that everything is a potential trigger. We have heard of people who are allergic to water, to air, to virtually all food items. The number of allergies, both in society and in individuals, augments in time. It appears as if the general trend is that one allergy leads easily to another, one trigger becoming two, three and so on. It seems clear that the problem does not lie with the trigger but with the individual's reaction to it.

Let's repeat the question of what an allergy is. An allergy is an over-reaction to some substance that the body registers as hostile. In the context of the body's survival mechanisms, this built-in defence reaction is entirely valid. Bodily resistance forms, amongst other things, antibodies against the allergens and this corresponds to a bodily defence reaction against hostile invaders which, from the body's point of view, is perfectly reasonable. In those who are allergic, however, this inherently sensible defence reaction is exaggerated out of all proportion. A high level of defence is built up, while the "hostile" category is extended to cover an ever-greater area. More and more substances are identified as "enemies" and the defence armoury is therefore increasingly strengthened in order to counter an increasing variety of enemies effectively.

Allergies and awareness

Here are two more interesting facts:

- Allergies always need consciousness as a condition for their appearance. There are no allergies under narcosis, and equally, all allergies fade away during psychosis. People suffering from Multiple Personality Disorder have certain allergies in one personality that disappear instantly when they take on a different personality.

- Illustrations of the allergen or pictures indicating conditions in which there would be a high exposure to a certain allergen can give rise to attacks in asthmatics and hay fever sufferers. In these experiments it is clearly demonstrated that the allergic reaction is totally independent of the presence of the allergic substance itself but is dependent on the state of mind of the individual.

These facts should help us to realise that allergens do not operate directly on the physical, chemical level.

What turns a body that is working well into an allergic wreck?

As life is energy and the body is energy that condenses as it materialises, why would an allergic reaction be anything else but an energetic interaction? If it were, this would immediately explain those observations where the physical trigger is not even present when a reaction occurs. It appears as if the mind, anticipating an offensive substance or situation, can trigger a physical reaction by itself. From this we could deduce that it is the mind that is extremely afraid of an outside situation, of particular energetic information in the environment. It knows it cannot cope and it is trying to avoid confrontation. It seems to know it has little defence against this information and would rather runaway than have to face the music. The fact that allergies, by and large, occur later in life indicates that these mind reaction patterns are a "learned" way to respond to such an environment.

Why? What can be so difficult about, for instance, pollen in springtime?

It is about the energetic message the environment is carrying. It is a time of renewal, time to get started again after winter, to rejoice and be jolly. However, waking up from your relatively dormant state requires energy, and you will need to put some effort into that process. Ask yourself whether your mind is happy to do so. Remember what it was like as a child, perhaps as a baby, to have newfound energy and drive. How did your parents respond to this yearly event of new life in the garden and in nature in general? Was it more of a nuisance, too much work, an unwelcome distraction? What kind of messages surrounding the situation did you grow up with?

The same questions can be asked about all over-sensitivity reactions. What is it really about? What was the feeling that triggered the physical response? Of course, most of the time the initial answer will be "nothing". We are not used to observing our lives in that way but, given a bit of practise and by learning to focus the mind again and again on looking beyond the physical, will soon deliver you some ideas and thoughts that will turn out to be useful in understanding your bodily responses to energetic information in general. It is in this way that you will discover real answers to the fear the mind has developed. This will allow you to stop the mind becoming more and more fearful about an increasing number of things. An allergic reaction or an over-sensitivity reaction is an expression of a fearful mind.

Overcoming allergies

How can you get rid of allergic reactions?

◄ Your mind's only task is to keep you alive. It will try and keep the system in balance under all circumstances for as long as it can. If it becomes afraid of certain circumstances, it means it has serious doubts about whether it can deliver on that promise. The reason it becomes very difficult or almost impossible to maintain balance is that it has become weighed down at one end of the scale. In life terms, that means there is too much ballast to carry and the mind is unable to lose it.

Too much ballast means it is high time to stop doing what you are doing and to concentrate on off-loading some excess baggage. It is time to stop. Stop everything. Take time off to be ill. No more work. No more socialising. No more chores. No more thinking. No more eating. Just rest, physically as well as mentally. Put your life on hold and allow your mind to direct energy to wherever it is required the most. It knows best. Allow the internal clean-up to take place.

While that is happening without you needing to put any attention towards the process you are free to contemplate what got you into this mess. Have a think about how far back in your life your system started having an aversion to certain things and situations. Collect data from various parts of your life and concentrate, not on the triggers for the allergic reactions, but on the circumstances in relation to stress, being pressured, feeling unfree. Within that data there is a common feature, a thread connecting the events. This may not be obvious to you. If it isn't then don't go forcefully looking for it. Sit with the observations and wait for the answer to come to you. It will become clear how deeply some of these conflict situations are rooted in your system, so be patient.

In the meantime, every time you find your allergic reactions getting worse again, simply take time off to be ill. Start to fast and to retreat from your ordinary life. Just a few days will give your system some more breathing space. Once the realisation about what the real underlying problem is emerges, you can put all your energy into making necessary changes in your life. Then your system will no longer be afraid, and you can become free. Don't be surprised if the changes that are required are fundamental to your old life and necessitate uprooting aspects of it. If the thread that triggers a serious allergic reaction is not life threatening, your system wouldn't panic in such a way. An allergic reaction bad enough to steer your life away from specific conditions and situations must have a life-threatening undertone. Once you have come to realise what that is, and only then, will you have the choice to free your life from the threat that may have been around for a large part of your life.

Here are a few words on allergies in babies and small children. They can suffer from stress too. Their inner life may struggle to find a decent foothold in their family. In order to fulfil the needs of a baby or a toddler we should not be looking into books on what's best for the child. We should be looking at the child in order to identify their needs. That will be very different for each child in the same household, so there cannot be a rule about all children being the same. A small child's serious allergic reaction is a message saying they feel very threatened in that household in this specific situation, under these specific conditions. If you, as a parent or grandparent, want to help such a child then get to know them better. Don't try and impose what you believe to be right but feel the inner life of the child. You may have to make fundamental changes to the child's environment and household, in order for the child's allergic reaction to disappear.

In general terms, a very young child lives by and in the energetic field of the household, of the parents, siblings and anybody else who is an integral part of daily life there. When a child becomes seriously or chronically ill it means there is imbalance in their life. As it is living its life through the energy field of its environment it is only by changing the environment that the child will be able to find its balance once again. The reason for a child being seriously ill lies in its environment. This is not about "good" or "bad". It is about the environment, at that time, being "right" for the child. That means determining whether the environment feeds the child's life in full or hinders their development. If the child is seriously ill, the answer is invariably "no". Each child has its own needs and they do not always fit in nicely with the adult's wishes and needs. In teenagers this will lead to clashes and be expressed in conflicts. Younger children don't have that ability to the same extent and tend to internalise conflicts, so they remain hidden from view. Then expression may become be chronic and serious illnesses may result.

You said that any substance is potentially an allergen, but there are certain substances that affect many more people and seem to be more likely to be triggers. These include gluten, crustaceans, eggs, peanuts and milk. Do you have an explanation for this?

What people in general overreact to is what they are increasingly exposed to. Exposure means two things, physical contact and mental exposure. When we encounter substances, nature does not know and that are difficult to handle, at some point we will reach our limit and our system will warn us. This is what is happening with the modern overuse of chemicals. Increasingly unnatural processes invade us. I include refining and processing food. Cleaning and disinfecting our environment is another process. However, most of the allergic reactions we are seeing are because people are being bombarded with "information" about the dangers of certain products. This causes a certain attitude of fear that leads to many more "cases". Even if most people are not really allergic to these substances, they end up being so fearful of them that they avoid contact, wishing to be "better safe than sorry" and thereby reducing the flexibility of their systems. They may become really rigid in these respects. In nature, allergies are extremely rare. However, in human culture they are an increasing problem. Is it to be assumed that there is something wrong in nature? No. Even though your system might manifest an overreaction in nature, that overreaction could be warning you that you have reached your limit of a particular substance. That reaction is not going to endanger your life. On the contrary, will probably save it.

You say that the number of allergies and allergens is increasing. Is this really the case? Is it known whether in the past there were few or no allergies? For example, I remember my mother telling me there were always children "allergic" to their mother's milk. Isn't that really extreme?

☙ Yes, there have always been allergic reactions in humans. There have always been serious warning signals from individual people's systems about their environments. Some children, it's true, are allergic to their mother's milk, but not to *all* mother's milk. They are clearly expressing an allergic reaction to their own mothers! They don't want their mothers to feed them because they are "energetically poisoning them". It is an energetic exchange, the experience a child has brought into the world with them, a message received from her mother during gestation. It is the only way she knows her mother.

Are you saying that any problem from the child's environment is expressed in an allergy or illness. Are all children's illnesses, including the most serious, related to the environments in which they live? What about children who are born with an illness? Is that also induced by the environment in which they live? What applies in pregnancy?

☙ We are all, and to an even greater extent very young children, "nurtured" by our environments. And yes, all chronic childhood diseases are caused by environments. Very young children absorb information from their environment directly, without filters through which they can choose what to believe. I explained this in one of the lessons of the course "Looking for Truth in Medicine" that we recorded at the Plural-21 Association in 2020. If you are interested, you can find it online.[5] There, I explain that the process of "poisoning" may have already started during gestation. It is not so much a physical poisoning, but rather an exposure to certain energies that the new human being struggles to fit into its own structure. Let's say that the information that it is receiving is unsettling the child, causing an imbalance in his life.

Are paediatricians and geriatricians needed?

You are very interested in the health of the youngest children, and you have done some research. What are your opinions on the existence of doctors specialising in children and babies, paediatricians. Is there a need for such specialisation? Are illnesses different in children and adults? What about specialists for older people, geriatricians?

➛ Paediatricians are a relatively recent addition to the medical profession. It is interesting to know that they use testing methods and therapies derived from adult medicine. There have been almost no studies done on the effects of any of the drugs used for infants and very young children. Their reasoning is that, because children suffer from the same illnesses as adults, whether they be cancer, arthritis, diabetes, epilepsy, or whatever, the same drugs must be appropriate for them. That is an assumption. They act and then observe the results of applying what are known to be toxic drugs. Their evaluation starts with the conviction that they are doing the right thing and so that anything that goes wrong is "bad luck" or something they "could not have known". They may use explanations such as saying a child already had a congenital abnormality that was not known, and which only appeared later in the disease process.

Geriatrics is also a new addition to medicine. Since medical authorities have taken over the care of the elderly, there has been

---

[5] https://timefortruth.es/2020/11/30/patrick-quanten-entrevistas-y-videos/

a lot more suffering and experimentation with drug protocols and surgical procedures.

Going back to allergies, you frequently talk about "defensive reactions", "antibodies", "defensive states" and "immune reactions". I have been wanting to ask you about this since the beginning of the book, and I think the time has come. Is there such a thing as an immune system? What is studied in immunology? Where is the immune system located? Is there indeed a defence system?

It is true that we use these terms very lightly. The plain truth is that there is no such thing as an "immune system". There is no separate set of organs responsible for defending the body, nor is one necessary. Life consists of continuous energy exchanges. Health is about maintaining an energetic balance within a given structure. This means that energy, a combination of frequencies, must remain within certain limits. When energy exceeds those limits, i.e. goes out of the range of comfort for that system, the energetic system of that organism struggles and its balance is disturbed. The person becomes ill.

"Maintaining balance" is the ability to move a little to the left or to the right whenever necessary. Therefore, the ability to maintain balance is related to one's personal ability to "absorb" disturbing energies without suffering harm. Thanks to the flexibility of the person's energy system, they can stay healthy. Such an ability is of vital importance, otherwise, anyone could, for example, die simply by getting wet. The environment changes all the time, and any living creature must have the ability to adapt to these changes. Thus, every cell and every system within each cell has a "natural range". Each set of organs within an organism has a natural range. There is no "defence" organ or system in the body. Staying healthy is simply being able to remain flexible throughout life. This, of course, becomes a little more difficult as we get older, as all our tissues lose some flexibility.

Many people would be perplexed to hear that there is no immune system. Today, the immune system is on everyone's lips: doctors, virologists, immunologists, scientists, politicians, the media (though I would label that as disinformation) and people in the street. Everyone is talking about the immune system and the whole world agrees that we have to keep our "immune systems" on high alert. Actually, it's funny that everyone is talking about something that doesn't exist. Do you think we could talk about the systems in the body that do exist?

�‒ Sure. Fortunately, there will always be people interested in knowing the truth.

Dogmatics

Dogmatics succeeded the two above-mentioned sects. [...]

It is certain that, to those who consider the order established by the Dogmatists for the study of this Art, it seems at first sight that it could not be more rational, because it recognises no other guide than natural philosophy.

Galen, authorising himself with the doctrine of Hippocrates, was the one who achieved a greater following than any other; and it is still enough to be a follower of his to achieve the credit of a great physician.

Such is the reputation and fame that his writings have had, that it is enough to quote a text of his to justify any murder, and for the greatest folly to be canonised. [...]

The entire complaint is against those who still want to obstinately defend their errors; for if Galen and Hippocrates were to come into the world again, they would be the first to erase themselves from their books and, without shame, they would learn many things that they were not fortunate enough to know in their own times.

They would not have written many things, if they had not held them to be true; which, apart from this, if they had then known the deception that was to follow, they would with the same zeal have condemned their own faults as they impugned those of others.

Yesterday and Today.
El mundo engañado por los falsos medicos
Extract from the book

IX

THE SEVEN SYSTEMS OF THE HUMAN BODY

Please talk about the systems that make up the human body. The classification of the various systems you use is not the same as in the anatomy books. It is interesting for me to discover how the body can be understood in such different ways.

◆ That's right, our classification is different. It is based on creation and the operational mechanisms of this evolutionary process. As different energies unfold throughout creation, the different corresponding physical manifestations are generated. One of the fundamental manifestations in living beings is the different bodily systems.

The most striking difference from the way in which the medical profession has divided up the body is the non-existence of an immune system. In the creative process there is no "immune system". Believe it or not, that corresponds to the general definition of "immunity". Immunity is the ability to maintain health and to resist disease. By this point in the book, you know you are not going to get sick as long as you manage the balance in all parts of your body well. The more balanced each of these parts are, the more resilient you will be against disease. In other words, immunity has nothing to do with an army heroically defending every cell of your body. Immunity doesn't need an army of its own. It only requires that every part of the body is in the best possible shape. Each cell "knows" what is best for it and, when it can achieve this, it is immune to disease.

Western medicine estimates that we have twelve systems in the body. You speak of only seven. I am intrigued to know what these seven systems are.

See the creation code and the consequences described in *Why Me? – Science and spirituality as inevitable bed partners*, written by me and Erik Bualda. Let's start with the notion from ancient wisdom that explains that there are seven types of tissue, that they originate one after the other and that each of them manifests from the previous one. This is explained in more detail in Chapter 2, "*How Life Works*". In the organism there are seven different tissues, and the order in which they appear is: water tissue (lymph), blood tissue, muscle tissue, fat tissue, bone tissue, nerve tissue and germ tissue. As we go down the list of tissues, each one is denser than the previous one and, at the same time, more complex.

Start from the notion in biology that every cell has the same structures as the whole body. In other words, from the first cell a complex organism will be constructed but all the information about what that structure will be is already present in a single cell. This should be no surprise as each seed holds all the information about the entire organism that will sprout from it. In essence we can say that every cell must therefore have the seven different tissues already in it, albeit in microscopic form.

Another very important point to understand is the basic physiology of creation. The first line of creation since the initial event that started our universe is a cooling down of the energetic fabric of the universe. This leads to a continually increasing pressure on the field which, in parts of the universe, results in the formation of matter. First are extremely small particles, atoms. Soon these are pushed together under the increasing pressure and form molecules, then more complex molecules and eventually "tissues". The number of basic tissue structures that can manifest? can be no more than the number of different energies present in the universe. The seven basic energies gradually become denser and follow a specific manifestation order. The densities increase as we move down the line. This is the order in which all manifestation within the universe occurs:

energy 1

energy 4

energy 6

energy 2

energy 5

energy 7

energy 3

The numerical figures correspond to the frequency bands these energies belong to, which is also manifested in the splitting of white light in its various colours, each with its own frequency band:

1 red

2 orange

3 yellow

4 green

5 blue

6 indigo

7 violet

This is in order of frequency bands. From 1 through to 7 there is a continual frequency change. The order 1-4-6-2-5-7-3 is the order in which these frequencies manifest within the universe, getting more and more dense and compact as the frequencies unfold and manifest. This is a direct result of the forces that are responsible for creation. Increasing pressure squeezes matter together more and more. There comes a point at which the particles making up matter can no longer be pushed together further but the pressure on matter still keeps increasing. At this point in creation a new format for tissues joining together appears. This is a cell. There is movement inside the cell. It is able to adjust to pressure. In fact, it can respond to pressure by splitting into two cells. Then the increasing pressure on the tissues no longer compacts the tissues, but spreads out the tissue, allowing it to occupy the space of two cells. This is the beginning of multiple cell organisms on earth.

If the organisms are a *blown up* version of the primary cell then it stands to reason that the organism will be made up in the same way as the original seed cell. The whole organism has the same characteristics as the primary cell. A corn seed can only produce corn and an acorn can only grow into an oak tree. A chicken egg can only produce a chicken, and no other bird or animal. All of this proves that the manifestation of the organism can be seen merely as a spread out version of the original seed cell. The seed cell must contain all the characteristics of the entire adult organism.

With seven basic energy forms in the field, only seven types of physical manifestation can be the result of increasing pressure. This means only seven basic tissues are found in any living cell and that these seven tissues must give rise to the visible structure of the organism. It is very likely that the manifestation of these structures develops over time and manifests in various organisms as creation rolls along. Various living organisms will still be around, or have been around, in which specific structures are most noticeable, even though all seven tissues are present to some extent within every living cell. Not all will manifest in every detail, nor will all organisms display the full range of potential of each of these seven tissues. It is, as creation itself, a gradual process of manifestation. But what is it exactly we are looking for?

Each of the seven primary tissues should develop into one macroscopic part of the body. This is true whether we are 'talking about a mollusc or a human being. We are considering the seven vital systems in an organism as related to the seven tissues that are vital for life.

1 – Watery tissue

Water is present in all organisms. It makes up the largest part of any organism and is in human beings organised as the *lymphatic system.*

4 – Blood tissue

There is definitely a lot of blood tissue within the human body, and it is organised in the *circulatory system.*

6 – Muscle tissue

The main characteristic of muscle tissue is the potential for contracting and releasing. This creates a pumping effect and then movement, but initially this system can only move very light material. At this stage of creation these are gases (atoms and light molecules) and simple molecules (sugars, fats and proteins). These are the *breathing and digestive systems*, two different aspects of the same principle. Breathing exchanges gases, oxygen and carbon dioxide. and the digestive system exchanges water and molecules of solid food) with the environment of the organism. The apparent split between these two separate systems can be traced back to the energetic field at this level, as the subdivision of frequency 6 has two possibilities of manifestation. The two possibilities deliver very similar systems as the differences only occur in the frequencies that are the least prominent in these systems (frequencies 7 and 3).

2 – Fat tissue

The main characteristic of fat is the fact that it is a tissue that stores energy. It is therefore a source of energy for any organism, a vital part of surviving. As organisms evolve mobility becomes a real manifestation towards more freedom, greater autonomy and better chances of survival. survival chance. This is the *mobility system*.

5 – Bone tissue

This is not so obvious. However, there is a system within any organism that lies in between the mobility and the yet to develop *nervous system*. This is a system that becomes necessary once an organism begins to move around and use its mobility to increase its survival chances. This system is a step towards the nervous system as that is the next system to follow, originating from this system and lying between fat tissue and nervous tissue. To make more efficient use of mobility we need to take more notice of the environment. More information needs to be gathered, processed and stored for this growth process to continue. This tissue manifests as the *sensory system*.

7 – Nervous tissue

This is a simple one as nervous tissue has become organised in the *nervous system*.

3 – Seed tissue

This, of course, is the procreation system. However, let's take a closer look at procreation. The entire operation is about glands and the interaction of hormones which are specific proteins. As there are glands in all the other systems apparently without those glands being able to reproduce anything as seeds do, it may be wise to take another look.

It is quite easy to prove that glands do not produce the specific hormones and/or proteins and enzymes as we have been made to believe. Simple observation and deduction show us that glands take up material rather than releasing it. They are, in a sense, recycling factories, cleaning up the systems, thereby "reproducing" material time and time again. Glands break down waste material and offer the basic building blocks back to the system. In a sense, this is a "rebirth", which is the basic characteristic of a seed. A seed is capable of manifesting another specimen of the same kind. Glands are capable of allowing the organism to re-manifest without it first having to die. This tissue is the *glandular system*.

water tissue	lymphatic system
blood tissue	circulation system
muscle tissue	breathing/digestive system
fat tissue	mobility system
bone tissue	sensory system
nervous tissue	nervous system
seed tissue	glandular system

Before we go on to take a look at each of these systems in more detail, I would like to point out that there is no such thing as "an immune system".

Although the medical profession tries to "prove" immunity via a variety of different chemical and blood tests, none of their efforts have resulted in any reliable protocol. Immunity is the resistance an organism has for withstanding possible disease factors or resisting being ill. With all their testing and insistence on knowing how immunity translates into the physical body, clinicians still have to admit they come across people with very low "immunity" test results who do not fall ill. Other people have strong "immunity" test results and are constantly getting ill. You would have thought that intelligent doctors would have concluded that their tests are useless, but they haven't. They persist in using such tests as "standard proof" of immunity and continue to base their recommendations on them when they are promoting, for instance, vaccination programmes.

There is no immunity system and inside single cells there are no organelles performing "protective" tasks. There is no presence of an army patrolling the interior of the cell and killing off intruders. Resistance against disease is the capability to withstand being pushed out of balance. Disease is an imbalance of the system. When the system remains in balance in spite of changing circumstances it manifests a high degree of immunity, resistance. Each cell and system tries to maintain balance through using energetic interactions. When your radio set has a stable set of frequency bands it will hold a radio station very well, even under extreme atmospheric conditions. It is immune to a lot of influences from the atmosphere and the material structures on the way to your radio set. On the other hand, you may have an older model with more disturbances on frequencies, resulting in crackling and fading. That is an imbalance of the system.

Let's return and study in more detail the seven systems that do exist. Why waste time on one that doesn't? It is very important to realise that each system, no matter how different it is from the others, is made of the same seven tissues. A pig has the same seven systems as a human being, even though they are rather different. The difference is even more striking once you realise that even a goldfish has those same seven systems. It is not because the overall expressions are so different that they cannot be made out of the same building blocks. With my lego blocks I can build a house, a car, a horse or anything else but it is still made from the same stuff. To find out how these same tissues create seven different systems we need to revisit the energetic field.

From creation we know that every one of the seven major energy bands has been made up from a combination of the same seven frequencies. We know the exact way the combinations come together in the seven different bands. Combining the same frequencies in different quantities results in a different overall energy field. The quantities are fixed in nature by the Golden Ratio and as we move down the coding line the contribution lessens with each step according to a predetermined natural pattern. We can, from the Golden Ratio, calculate the percentage contribution of each step as we move down the line:

$$39.55906\% - 24.44888\% - 15.11025\% - 9.3386\% -$$
$$5.77156\% - 3.56707\% - 2.20455\%$$

Following the way energies manifest in creation, we can show the contributions of each frequency to each band:

FREQUENCY BANDS	FREQUENCY CODES	REMARKS
frequency 1	1-4-6-2-5-7-3	is also the Creation Code
frequency 4	4-6-1-2-3-5-7	
frequency 6	6-4-2-1-5-3-7 6-4-2-1-5-7-3	there are two possibilities
frequency 2	6-4-2-1-5-3-7 2-6-5-7-4-1-3 2-5-6-4-7-1-3 2-5-6-7-4-1-3	there are four possibilities
frequency 5	5-7-2-6-4-1-3	
frequency 7	7-5-2-6-4-1-3	
frequency 3	3-1-4-6-2-5-7	

For a visual picture you can see how they are made of the seven colours by replacing the figures with corresponding colours.

1 red – 2 orange – 3 yellow – 4 green
– 5 blue – 6 indigo – 7 violet

The seven tissues combine in various ways that result in seven different systems, together making up the whole organism. Let's look at the systems with their corresponding energy bands in more detail within the human form.

Frequency 1
The Lymphatic System (1-4-6-2-5-7-3)

This is the first system to develop in any multicellular organism. It basically consists of water and a "skin", a layer that separates the organism from the outside world. The largest tissue contributions to this system come from energy 1 (water tissue

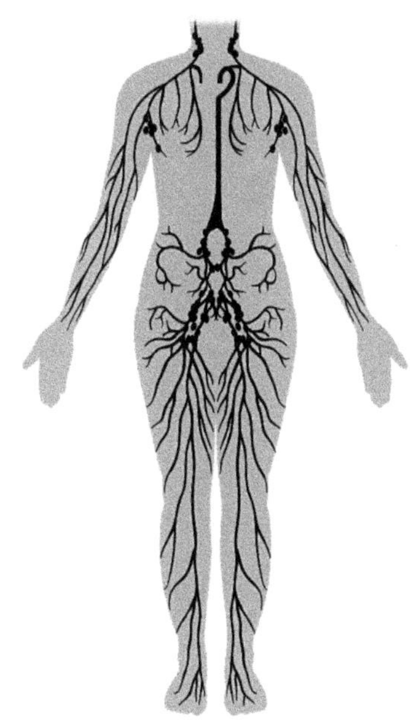

– 39.55906%), energy 4 (blood tissue – 24.44888%) and energy 6 (muscle tissue – 15.11025%). Blood tissue is in essence a thickening of water, whereby water carries heavier materials (proteins and fats). Muscle tissue provides contraction, which allows water to be pushed forward, thereby creating movement. As you can see from the code of this system, there is, in the last position, also a contribution of energy 3 (2.20455%), which is tissue that manifests as glands. In the lymphatic system, glands only occupy about 2.2% but this is just as essential as water as it is integral to the balance of the system and the way it functions. These glands filter and clean the water flowing from the cells, removing cellular debris.

The lymphatic system provides the basic living conditions for any organism, no matter how complex. Flowing water containing substances forms the basic harmonious ecosystem between an organism and its outside world. It forms the first exchange system between inner and outer world.

As organisms develop further, the next system will manifest in the lymphatic system and become a separate unit. As Ayurveda teaches us, each tissue, and in due course each subsequent system, emerges from within the previous existing system.

Frequency 4
The Circulatory System (4-6-1-2-3-5-7)

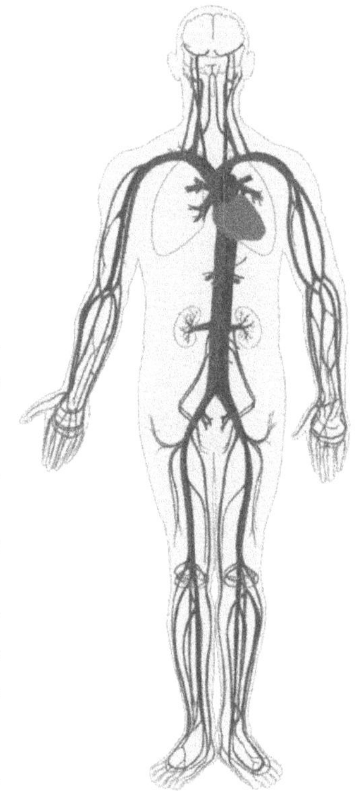

The circulatory system exists within the "water system" but becomes a separate system whereby blood can run in separate vessels. Separation is clear because each system has its own "skin", its own membrane. Here this is blood vessel walls. The main components of the circulatory system are blood tissue (4), muscle tissue (6) and water tissue (1). The large majority of the circulatory system consists of muscular tubes (arteries and veins) pushing forward water (plasma) and various blood cells (blood tissue). However, as in all systems, there are other components that make up a balanced system. Energy 3 has a larger role to play, resulting in a greater presence of glands in the circulatory system. There are the kidneys (filtering and cleaning the water element in the blood), spleen (filtering and cleaning up damaged and old blood cells) and the thymus (cleaning up white blood cells).

Blood tissue emerges from the previous tissue layer, which is the lymphatic system, the water tissue. There is a constant exchange of material between the two systems. Nutrients as well as waste products flow via the lymphatic system into the circulation and vice versa. Nutrients feed and empower the cells of the circulatory system, while waste products are eliminated by the glands. The glands break down and recycle basic materials, releasing them back into circulation as basic nourishing or building structures, from where they are also offered back to the cells of the lymphatic system.

The next level of creation will emerge from the previous one, which is the circulation system, the blood tissue.

Before we continue, I am curious. What is the function of the heart in the circulatory system? Is it just to pump blood?

-❧ No, blood is pumped throughout the body by the contraction and relaxation of the pumping function of the blood vessels, the arteries. The heart is the control centre, in a similar way as the brain is for the nervous system. The heart sets the rhythm, the rhythm of life. It responds to stimuli from the environment by changing the rhythm. That is why we relate feelings to the heart. The rhythm of the heart determines our peace, anxiety, fear, frustration, anger and so on. I have a mental picture of this. It goes back to historical ship building. These ships were propelled by oarsmen on both sides. The pace at which they rowed, as well as signals for left and right, were set by a man pounding a drum.

Frequency 6
Digestive and Respiratory Systems
6-4-2-1-5-3-7, called 6A
6-4-2-1-5-7-3, called 6B

At this energetic level, a split occurs and consequently two different, but closely related systems emerge. Both systems, separated from each other by their own membranes and from every other system, are mainly constructed out of muscle tissue (6), blood tissue (4) and fat tissue (2). In the digestive system we find that the digestive tubes (oesophagus, stomach and gut) are mainly made up of muscles, which is also the case with the blood vessels in this system. Besides this, there is a large fat content in the digestive tract cells, and right through to the accompanying glands. Similarly, in the breathing system there is a large muscle tissue content in all the alveoli, the small balloons in the lungs that blow up and contract, in the trachea and in every further division of the lung pipes, not forgetting the large number of blood vessels that run through the lungs. This confirms the presence of an enormous amount of blood tissue, whilst the optimal functioning of the alveoli requires the constant presence of fat tissue.

The structure of these systems is very similar. From the central tubes a massive network of blood vessels connects everything, from the digestive part to the cleaning station glands and from the breathing part to the heart. Both show clearly how they have emerged from the previous one, the circulatory system. In a sense they each "hang" at the end of a large tree of blood vessels. Hence both systems exchange information, energy and matter, with the circulatory system.

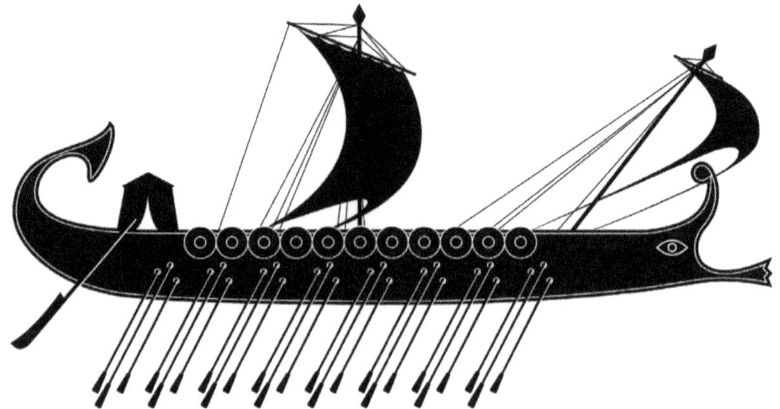

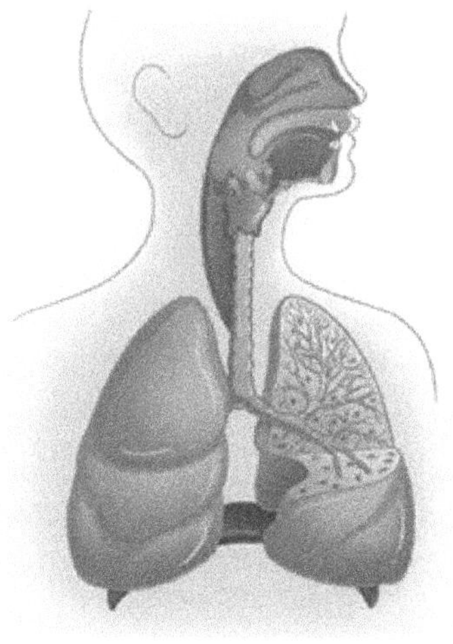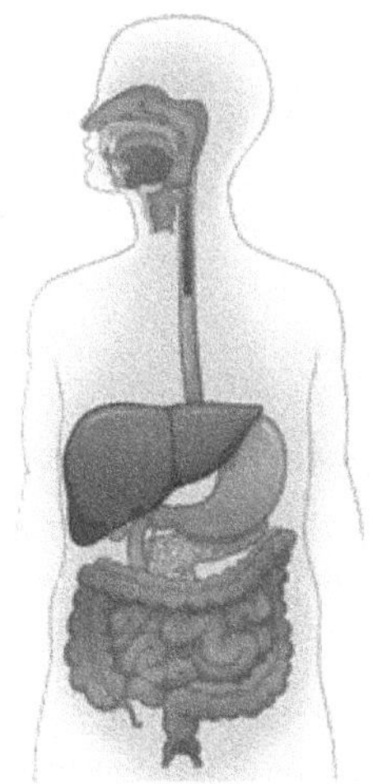

In the digestive system, solid heavier materials are being taken into the cells of the upper section and heavier waste material is being expelled by the cells in the lower section. In contrast, respiration happens on the level of gases, very light matter. Here cells in contact with outside gases take in gas molecules to fuel cells and release waste gas. The first obvious manifestation of this two-part system in creation is the occurrence of larger plants. The root systems of plants (energy 6A) exchange matter with the earth and the leaves of the plants (energy 6B) with the atmosphere. From then on this dual system is a feature of all organisms that follow on.

Energy 6B ends its code on frequency 3, indicating the emergence of a new development in that energy field. It is like the seed of a new beginning. Up to this point of development, including in the digestive system, every system emerged *inside* the previous system. The respiratory system breaks this mould and emerges *outwardly*. In the digestive tract we see how the digestive cells in the oesophagus, stomach and gut lie at the end of blood vessels, so that the circulatory system is encircling the digestive tract. In the respiratory system, however, the blood vessels "open up" to the atmosphere. They do not enclose the system but are open ended.

To get a picture of the contribution of the less obvious tissues in these systems we will take a look at the presence of glands (3).

There are more glands, and they play a more significant role in the digestive part as compared with the respiratory part. Glands that are directly connected with the digestive system and are lying inside its membrane, are the liver, gallbladder and pancreas. The respiratory system only has submucosal glands to keep the epithelium of the tubes and alveoli moist and to clean the surfaces.

From now on new emerging systems will still arise from within the previous existing ones but will develop outwardly. This leads to systems extending beyond the boundaries of the internal cavities, the abdomen and chest.

Frequency 2

The Motor System

2-6-5-4-7-1-3, called 2A

2-6-5-7-4-1-3, called 2B

2-5-6-4-7-1-3, called 2C

2-5-6-7-4-1-3, called 2D)

In the energetic field there are four possibilities. These are expressed in matter, in the structure and function of the motor system. The motor system develops in four stages, working its way out of the core. Early animals such as worms and snakes moved with contractions of their circular bodies. Then, during the universal manifestation of energy 2, more free movement was first achieved through the use of fins, as in fish. This developed further in amphibians, when the pelvic area (frequency 2) and the corresponding shoulder area (frequency 5, second in the coding system for 2) grew extensions. These extensions allow movement on land as well as in the sea. On land the motor system develops further into the four footers, from salamanders into reptiles, where the front and hind legs work in conjunction to provide movement, and into birds. In birds, there is a distinctly different use for the extensions of the pelvis from the use there is for the shoulders. The fourth development of mobility is walking on two hind legs as seen only in primates

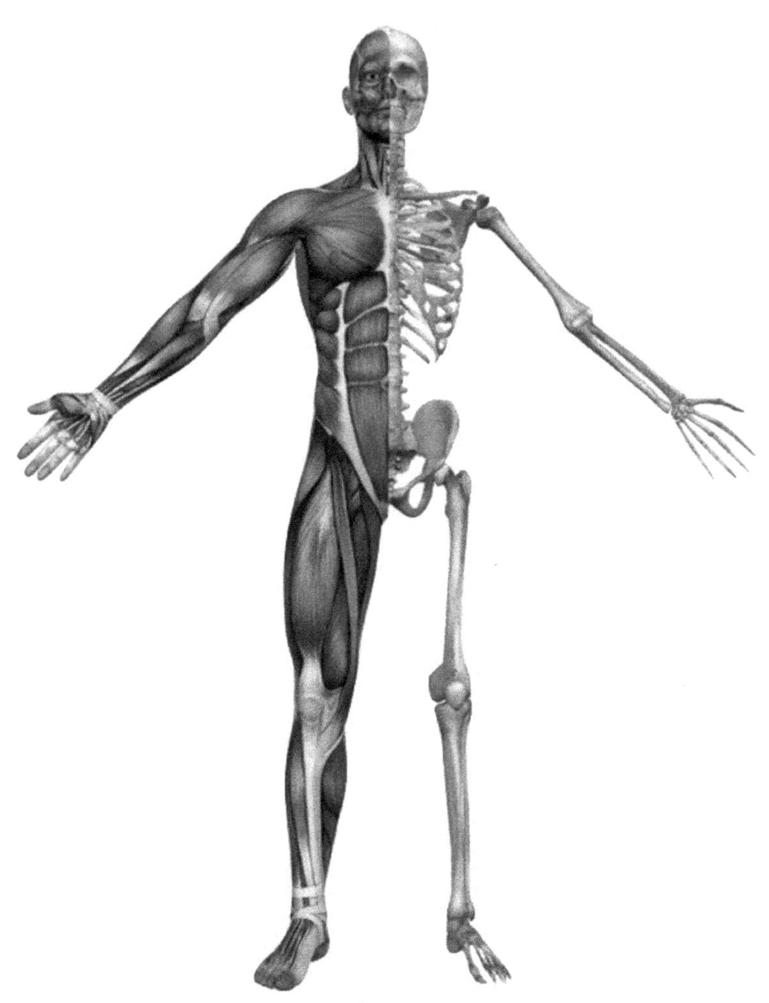

including humans. First there are fins, then four footers, then birds and then walking upright. The motor system is mainly made out of fat tissue (2), muscle tissue (6) and bone tissue (5). When we talk about the motor system in human beings, we need to consider mainly the arms and legs as the development specific for the motor system. Of course, any structure with muscle tissue will move but this is all about the way the organism as a whole creates mobility for itself. Humans no longer use the spine as much for movement, but our bodies have specially designed features that correlate to the kind of movement that is appropriate for us.

Energy 3 is as the smallest contribution in all codes for the energy band 2 placed, in the last position. What glands does the motor system use? Movement depends on fat tissue (2) and muscular contraction (6). The more contractions the body requires the more fat it needs to burn up and the more waste products those contractions leave behind. This means the body needs to have adapted by creating a clean-up system of glands to deal with the waste. The motor system mainly depends on the adrenal glands and the thyroid gland. With the development of the motor system we can also, for the first time in evolution, clearly distinguish seven parts in the one system. These seven subdivisions are present in all systems, but it isn't as clear how we can distinguish them, for instance, in the lymphatic system. In the motor system we can identify the seven parts of the one system, mainly because the movement hinges on a solid structure, the skeleton, that allows powerful muscular contractions. That kind of movement requires limbs, and it is through those that we can see the seven-part structure of the skeleton.

1. Tail
2. Pelvis and lumbar region – hips – legs
3. Transition lumber to thoracic region
4. Thoracic back
5. Shoulder blades – shoulders – arms
6. Neck
7. Skull

Frequency 5
Sensory System (5-7-2-6-4-1-3)

This follows on from the development of the motor system that allows more diverse mobility. With this comes the need for a good system to sense the environment as the organism moves around.

Once again, this system develops within the previous one, confirming the trend in moving outwardly. Our well-developed sensory organs are located in the bony structure (5), the skull, because this is an extension of the more primitive nervous system of earlier animals. Never lose sight of the fact that all animals have sensory organs, but here we are talking specifically about their refining through various developmental stages. We can see from the coding that the main contributions are made by bone tissue (5), nervous tissue (7) and fat tissue (2). Indeed, all sensory organ activity will require a lot of energy, which explains the input of frequency 2.

How does a sensory organ work? We are told it "collects" information from the environment but that doesn't tell us exactly how or what kind of information it collects. We can already deduct and agree that the information collected is energetic. Sensory organs pick up light frequencies, sound frequencies, and smell frequencies so. let's be clear about their non-material function. This level of development puts non-matter over matter. Now for the question of how an organ selects which frequencies to picks up. Let me make two observations. Firstly, each sensory organ picks up frequencies within a specific range (visible light, sound and smell). Secondly, at any given moment two people in the same spot do not receive the same signals. Sometimes one person sees or smells something that the other person cannot. This is important to understand if we want to understand how these organs work.

Before you can pick up any specific frequencies from the entire spectrum available in the outside world you need to send out a "question". The sensory organs first send out messages and then pick up the "replies" from the environment, rather like radar. Bats navigate like that. Here is the secret. We do too! It is, in fact, the only way to be in the environment. Doctors will confirm that some people born blind will have perfectly formed eyes, leaving them to speculate on whether the nervous system is not working properly and is therefore responsible for their blindness. The reason for their blindness is the fact that the organ is not sending out a message. Everything is ready and functional for receiving the incoming information but if no question is being asked, no answer can be forthcoming.

The sensory organs send out frequencies, each within a specific band, allowing for the separation between vision, hearing, touch etc. In order to "feel" something the nerve supply to the area of that part of the body must be intact. Nerves move a signal through to the skin. This allows you to evaluate the part of the outside world you are in direct contact with via the information carried back. Your "expectations" of what you are touching will colour your evaluations. You may be shocked or may relax and enjoy. You will evaluate, note your experience and store the information. If you expect to touch a metal plate your nervous impulses will "prepare" for that, but when the plate turns out to be hot, or even just slightly warm, you'll pull back and have to re-arrange your nervous impulses in order to touch it again and get a more accurate sense of what that part of the outside world is like. Similarly, if you don't expect to see a snake you may simply see a fallen branch from a tree. If you are not paying attention because you don't expect a bird to sing, you may not hear it. You don't see what you are not paying attention to. Be careful to note that "attention" does not only mean conscious attention. Our nervous system has learned to pay attention to a lot of things we are no longer are conscious of but, because we have learned to always pay attention to that information, we do it automatically. This goes for all sensory organs. As these organs develop through various animal species, they become more sophisticated, but the principle remains the same.

The sensory organs, like all other systems, develop through the history of the universe and are expressed in various types of organisms. Therefore, each of the senses has to relate directly to a frequency band.

1 – sense of touch

4 – sense of vision

6 – sixth sense (intuition) – definitely works from the inside out.

2 – sense of hearing – in order to hear we must create sound and so there are two separate parts developed at this stage, voice and hearing

5 – sense of smell

7 – sense of taste – this is still being developed in human beings, apparently with a long way to go before completion

3 – sense of ? – this will develop during the next evolutionary stage, whatever comes after human beings, and I understand will be expressed through the sexual organs and relate to personal power.

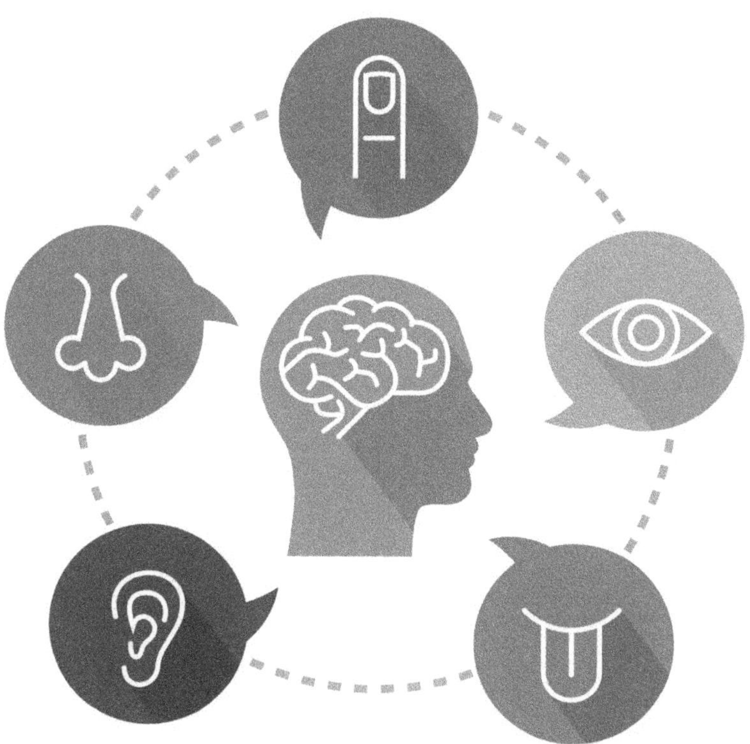

In each of the seven sensory organs we also find glands as indicated by frequency 3, present in the smallest amount as seen within the code of energy band 5. Some are more obvious than others, but they include tear production, earwax production, nasal secretions for smell and salivary glands for taste.

You say that sensory organs first send out a message and then pick up the "response" from the environment, as with radar. If no question is being asked, no response will follow. I wonder what happens to autistic children, assuming their bodies have stopped sending out signals because they are not interested in communicating with the environment. Why would an organism make such a decision?

➤ Autistic children, if we understand we are talking about real autism – children who have withdrawn from the world? send out fewer signals and they are of a specific nature. They are very attentive to certain signals, whereas they are completely ignorant of others. The reason for this is fear. They experience their environment as very threatening so they do not allow themselves to communicate with it. If you know you cannot win the argument, you stop trying. For most autistic children this process starts during foetal development. The origin can be traced back to the relationship between the baby, the mother and her environment, experienced by the foetus through her reactions to it. In most cases the mother is the one who best understands that her child has different needs. This may reflect the fact that, unconsciously, the mother is not happy with her environment or that there is a real rift within the family.

Frequency 7
The Nervous System (7-5-2-6-4-1-3)

The true potential of the nervous system will be developed in humans. As we are only at the beginning of this development in the universe, there is still a long way to go before it comes to fruition. We can see the outward movement of this system as nerves reach every part of the organism. They move towards all external parts in order to gather information but also to deliver information. The nervous system originates and matures within the sensory system, although it moves way out of the physical constraints of that manifestation. The sensory organs lie within the skull. The nervous system has its central part located there but part of the central nervous system, the spinal cord, develops outside of that restriction. Then the peripheral nervous system can be found everywhere in the body. The main contributors to this system are nervous tissue (7), bone tissue (5) and fat tissue (2). Compared to the previous system there is more nervous tissue and less bone tissue. Again, a lot of energy is used within this system, hence the presence of a lot of fat.

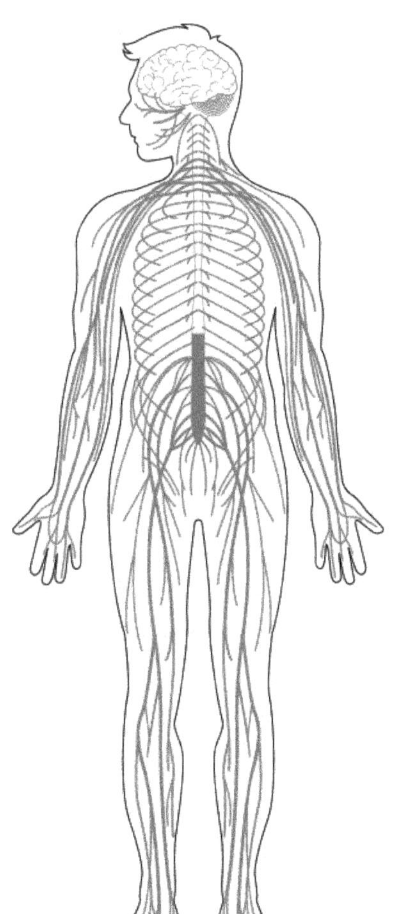

Glands, frequency 3, are present in the smallest possible number. They can be found inside the central nervous system in the brain, where they clean up waste products of nervous system activity, recycle it and return it to the cells.

Frequency 3
The Glandular System
(3-1-4-6-2-5-7)

This relates to seed formation and the sexual organs, in particular the glands, as they are the largest contributor to this system. The system will be fully developed during the next evolutionary stage of the universe, but it is, as it was with all other systems, a development from the previous one, in this case, the nervous system. Our sexual functioning depends greatly on our nervous system and our mental state. The glandular system consists mainly of glands (3), water tissue (1) and blood tissue (4). We can describe this in another way and say that seed (3) needs the right feeding ground (water and basic nutrition) to create new specimens. This is the ultimate *outgrowing* a system can achieve as it will, at this level, split into another specimen. The entire organism has outgrown itself.

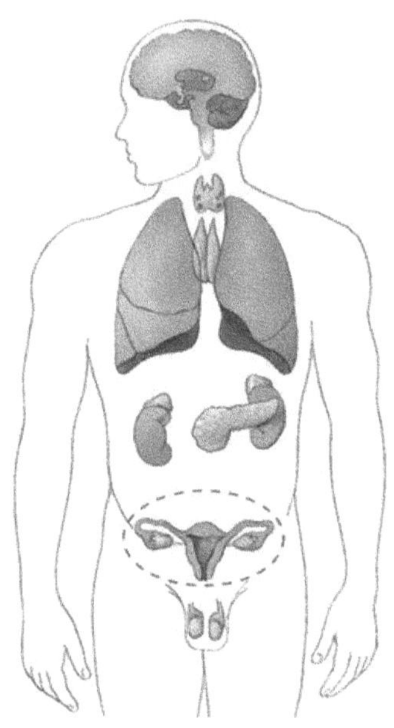

But Patrick, official medicine defines a gland as follows:

> **"A collection of cells whose function is to synthesise chemicals, such as hormones, to be released, often into the bloodstream and into a body cavity or its outer surface. These substances may be chemical messengers that are incorporated into the body to reach the cell for which they are destined, depending on their special characteristic, or to directly produce a specific effect on the medium into which they are secreted."**

However, when you spoke to us about the seed tissue, you defined glands in a quite different way as recycling factories that cleanse the system. In that way they "reproduce the system" over and over again, breaking down waste material and return building blocks back into the system. The glands absorb matter, rather than releasing it.

Those are two radically different options, don't you think? In the first definition, a gland secretes substances, hormones – and in the second, a gland recycles waste material. How is it possible that there are two such opposite views? Secondly, if the glands do not produce hormones, what does?

-❧ The glandular story, as told by the medical profession, makes no sense. It is based on the assumption that there is physical communication between different parts of the body. They ignore clinical scientific evidence because of the indoctrination they receive from industry. Science affirms that everything is energy, and that all communication is energetic exchange. Medical science itself has shown that the manufacture, transport and distribution of hormones, together with the time it takes for each cell to respond, cannot explain the rapid reaction patterns we see in life. In fact, the medical profession puts forward that the fastest communication system we have is the nervous system. This is much faster than the physical route they cling to in their story about hormones and glands, and yet they themselves realise that the fastest nerve pathway in the entire nervous system is about 100 times too slow to explain the speed at which the changes in the body occur during the fight or flight mechanism.

The only way to explain communication in the body is through frequencies, vibrations. An example is the thyroid gland, located in the neck. Venous blood samples taken from the arm show thyroid hormone levels on which doctors base their diagnoses and yet there are no thyroid glands in the arm or in the hand that could account for the production of these hormones! A common diagnostic test for the thyroid gland is photography with a technique called scintigraphy. This involves injecting radioactively labelled thyroid hormone into the bloodstream. After some time, the radioactive signal is detected *inside* the thyroid gland. Hence, the thyroid gland has absorbed the thyroid hormone from the bloodstream!

Forgive me for pressing the hormone issue. I still don't understand it. If the glands do not produce the hormones, what produces the hormones and what are they?

Hormones, as well as everything else cells need, are produced by the cells themselves. What each cell secretes is its own waste products. These "waste products" are what other cells use, what they need to live on. Hormones are the end products of internal cellular processes and are released as waste products of those processes. Each gland specialises in one type of waste and its cells feed on it. This stimulates the gland's activity. As a result of their metabolism these glandular cells release other waste products that will serve as food for other cells in the system. Everything is nothing more than a continuous cycle of recycling within the human ecosystem, a miniature sample of how nature itself works.

Ah, now I understand. It's fascinating, but it's also sad that the medical profession can't see it that way. What happens in a person's ecosystem when a doctor prescribes "artificial hormones"? Is he disrupting its balance?

Taking a hormone replacement treatment means altering someone's natural ecosystem. If there is a low blood level of a particular hormone, it means that the cells are not producing that hormone in large quantities. There has to be a reason for this, even if we don't understand why. This may indicate that the system is trying to maintain its balance by lowering the production of that hormone. Adding it artificially to the system stimulates the gland to clear out excess hormone. The gland will then work harder despite the naturally low production of the hormone within the system. The more artificial hormones are taken, the harder the system will have to work to reduce the hormone level it requires in order to maintain balance. The system will then further reduce the natural production of that hormone. This is how the vicious circle is perpetuated. My conclusion is that hormone replacement therapy does nothing but further reduce the natural secretion of hormones, and therefore only worsens the problem it is intended to solve. Instead of "curing" the low natural hormone production, what hormone replacement therapy does is to cause a reduction in the natural production of the hormone.

It is a simple and effective way of making sure that people become physiologically imbalanced and increasingly ill. At the time, nobody will notice what is happening, because everybody is just looking at blood levels of the hormone. Nobody is looking at how the organism as a whole works.

Among the seven systems you talked about are two dedicated exclusively to cleaning and recycling, the lymphatic system and the glandular system. In addition, in all the other systems there are also glands (energy 3) that cleanse. The human body, therefore, is a system which is in great need of cleansing in order to survive. Cleansing seems to be the most important activity of the organism!

◆ Indeed. Most failures of any system are directly related to an excess of waste. The same can be said with respect to the earth itself. The problem is not that there is a shortage of food. The problem is that consumer society produces too much waste. Throwaway culture and planned obsolescence have meant that we are drowning in our own waste.

Back to the human system, each of the seven systems is made up of cells. Cells are like factories that continually produce waste, as this is one end-result of metabolism. This needs to be dealt with first at a local level, the glandular cells in that system. However, when a particular system is required to work harder, for the good of the entire system, then the resulting extra waste must be removed from local cells and transported to the big recycling plants, the glandular system. The first objective of all glandular cells is to recycle. When there is overload, there will be excretion, disposal of waste from the body. For gaseous waste this will occur through the lungs, digestive system and skin. Liquid waste will be excreted through the kidneys, the intestine/upper respiratory system and the skin. Fat-soluble waste will be excreted via the intestine and skin. Good health therefore depends on effective waste management.

Conclusions

What does knowledge of these seven systems bring to understanding the healing process?

➤ Everything is made of energy, and it is through repetition of the same sequences that multiple manifestations come into being. When a frequency ceases to be harmonious, no longer fitting easily into its natural spectrum, this imbalance will manifest itself on all levels. For example, when frequency 2 becomes unbalanced it will alter the function, and later on even the structure of fatty tissue, but, at the same time there will be repercussions for the motor system. Frequency 2 is present in all systems and everywhere in the organism. Wherever the effect of any small imbalance manifests, it means that it is more noticeable in those areas than in other areas of the body, but the repercussions will be felt in all systems.

In more practical terms, what does this mean?

➤ It means that there will be malfunctioning in various parts of the body due to the imbalance of the same single frequency. All the signs, symptoms and expressions of an imbalance are related to each other and have a single energetic cause. For example, problems with the eyes, heart and circulation, breathing and/or digestion can all be expressions of a single problem in frequency 4.

Similarly, we can manifest the hardening of a specific tissue, a "tumour". This results from the condensation of one of the regular frequencies of energy. It manifests itself first in a system, the one in which that energy frequency is under the greatest pressure. If the pressure that is causing the condensation persists, then it stands to reason that the same energy frequency in another primary system manifests the same hardening in the same type of tissue, a hardening which we then call a "secondary tumour". This is explained by western medicine – above – as a cell from the primary tumour breaking off and traveling to another part of the body, where it begins to proliferate and form a new tumour similar to the primary tumour. No reason for this is ever given. As everything in life is energetic, the same imbalanced frequency that hardens its corresponding tissue, manifested in one part of the body, will in time, also condense the same tissue in another part of the body, A tumour is nothing more than a physical expression that tells us what is happening in the energetic field.

Therefore, gathering all the physical expressions, every little sign and symptom, will lead us to identifying which frequency is under pressure and why. This is the information needed before any healing can take place. The medical profession manages to make the population believe they are the health experts and that there is nothing more to know than what they know. That's why they tell you they don't know what the cause of your illness is. However, magically, they always have a treatment ready for you. When they think they know the cause, but their treatment doesn't work, they never consider that their analysis of cause and effect might be wrong. In the event a treatment doesn't work, the patient has simply had "bad luck".

Failure to compare and contrast results always underpins any established system. We all know that the medical industry spends a lot of time, money and effort on finding out what the public think of its products or services, but the medical profession has become so smug and arrogant that it has no need to know what its actions and treatments actually achieve. When you are comfortably settled on your ivory throne, you don't care about the plebs. That is a direct road to stupidity.

Existing systems according to medical science:

1. Digestive system: set of organs responsible for the process of digestion. It is made up of the oesophagus, stomach, small intestine and large intestine.

2. Nervous system: specialises in the transmission and processing of nerve signals. Includes the central nervous system. Consists of the cerebrum, cerebellum and spinal cord, and the peripheral nervous system, formed by the sensory and motor nerves.

3. Respiratory system: enables the exchange of gases with the environment. Its main organ is the lung.

4. Circulatory system: consists of blood, a set of ducts – arteries, veins and capillaries – and a driving pump, the heart.

5. Endocrine system: consists of all the organs and tissues that produce hormones. Hormones are chemical substances that are mainly transported through the blood and act on other cells to regulate their functions.

6. Bone system: consists of all the bones and cartilage that make up the human skeleton.

7. Muscular system: consists of the skeletal muscles. The sum of the muscular system plus the skeletal system gives rise to the locomotor system, which makes movement possible.

8. Excretory system: responsible for the production, storage and excretion of urine. It consists of the kidneys, ureters, urinary bladder and urethra.

9. Reproductive system: the sets of organs involved in sexual reproduction.

10. Immune system: provides the body's ability to distinguish its own cells and tissues from foreign cells and substances, and to neutralise or destroy the latter by different mechanisms, including the production of antibodies.

11. Lymphatic system: the system that transports lymph, an extracellular fluid.

12. Integumentary system: consists of the skin, nails, hair and
related glands. Its function is to protect the body with an insu-
lating layer that prevents infection and helps keep body temperature stable.

Do you want to know how easy it is to medicate oneself?
Observe that all animals are cured by the pure instinct of nature;
for as Cato wishes:
Sua cuique Natura est ad vivendum dux.
The Nature of each one is for that one the guide to life.
She is the first to facilitate the way and the means for its preservation.

Nor can I persuade myself that men lack this benefit.

Especially as I often see many sick people who,
abandoned by their doctors
and administering to them what they desire,
they have been relieved of those infirmities from which they were
oppressed.
They are stimulated by certain desires,
and when they have fulfilled them, they recover,
recognising in this their convalescence.

And is all this anything else but pure instinct,
or, to put it more correctly, the inspiration of nature
which makes them desire that which may be of relief to them?

Yesterday and Today.
El mundo engañado por los falsos medicos
Extract from the book

X

WORKING STRATEGIES
TO RESTORE HEALTH

I know you are not a great lover – not a lover at all, for that matter – of therapies in general, but I would like to offer readers some advice in relation to therapies. Can you recommend any? Do you think there are any that work?

✎ Do you want to know what I think about therapies? Therapies transfer your power to an external source. They transmit to the nervous system the message that you are powerless, that you are a helpless victim. The reality is that the best any therapy can do for you is to convey a message to your system. Therapies can influence your system, but not establish the change you need. Since "change" is the only real therapy, it is only the individual who can make the necessary changes and maintain them. Unfortunately, for almost two hundred years we have been living a big lie in the field of health. The medical profession is part of a scam created solely to turn people into addicts dependent on supposedly trained medical professionals. In reality they are nothing more than pawns of the industrial system. Nothing that is proposed or done by doctors in relation to illness can be of any use to anyone. To say something different or to leave the door open to the "possible" usefulness of such medical approaches to health is to deceive people even more. Personally, I refuse to do that any longer.

On the contrary, what we who are waking up to all this need to do is to educate people and to keep their minds focused on their own power, not diluting or watering down our message simply because the truth may be difficult for most people to assimilate. Those with these views may soon be faced with a difficult decision, either keeping quiet and fully complying with what we have been told, or being expelled from society. I want people to know they are in control of their own health and that they don't need the help offered by the medical authorities at all.

We do not want or need to offer people any therapy, and that includes homeopathy. As we have been pointing out, the authoritarian medical system doesn't work because health is an individual matter and therefore must be taken care of by an individual. All we can offer is the knowledge that the power is within you.

You mentioned homeopathy. Do you have anything to say about it?

◆ True homeopathic treatments are administered in single doses, which can be repeated at most one or two more times, with the intention of stimulating the energetic system to restore the existing imbalance. The homeopathic dose is directed towards the energetic frequency in which someone has problems. It is not a symptom-directed treatment if we are talking about true homeopathy. The same symptoms in different people will need different remedies. The remedy is for all the symptoms and irritations a particular person has at a particular time. There are no long-term treatments. Each treatment is the result of the assessment of the current time in that person's life and consists of administering the energetic frequency that is causing the problem. I repeat: there is no generalised and universal homeopathic treatment, but only individualised treatment for specific moments in people's lives.

More important than homeopathic treatments are homeopathic principles. It must be recognised that they are true expressions of natural laws:

- Like cures like. Using the same stimulus will "focus" the energy and increase its strength.
- Small amounts stimulate, large amounts obstruct. Using a small quantity will concentrate the energy and cause the body

to react to that incoming energy. The use of a large amount will result in a withdrawal of energy, as the body will try to "protect" itself against the excessive amount and will not be stimulated.

- Everything is connected and everything influences everything else.
- There is no physical exchange of anything, it is always a matter of exchanges and interactions between different energies.

What about fasting? I know for a fact that it is a therapy, technique or habit – that really works.

-🍂 Fasting is an essential part of any healing and is used as a first-line medical treatment in all traditional health systems. The reason for this is very simple: it is natural. Animals do it. Plants do it. Changing habits in order to prevent or cure a system from overloading takes time. Not "feeling well" is associated with a loss of appetite and a natural tendency not to eat. In all the world's civilisations, and throughout the centuries, we find traditions showing the human relationship with fasting. Instruction manuals for spiritual development in all religions include the advice to fast regularly. Fasting is natural. Fasting is fundamental. And yet, the experts of the Western medical system tell us it is dangerous, that it will make us sick and that we can even die from it. Funny, isn't it? You have two choices: either you believe in something that mankind, along with the rest of nature, has always used successfully, or you believe in those who take advantage of your need to regain your health and who are employees of the industry.

Fasting has an effect on the entire system, physical and mental. On the other hand, the more food we eat, the more food we need. Our systems like routine. If there is plenty of food around, our systems need constant confirmation that the abundance is still there, still available. The more we eat, the hungrier we get! Our mental focus on food leads us to believe we need it all the time. We depend on food and on the abundance of food. However, everything entering the body must be processed, broken down and recycled. Thus, the more we eat, the more work we demand from our system. The busier our system is digesting, the less energy it has available for anything else.

Stopping the cycle of dependency, the idea that we need something all the time in order to survive, is achieved by fasting. You must stop eating to experience feeling you don't need food all the time in order to live. You have to stop eating to experience the true feeling of energy and clarity.

Fasting gives us the opportunity to break many habits. This is fundamentally beneficial to our health because it stops the continuous accumulation of waste products in our systems. These waste products are the end result of the burning that releases energy in cellular activity. If we use less energy, we provide our cells with more space and time to carry out other jobs as well. In addition, fasting allows us to divert our attention from our daily routines related to food to other things. It gives us space and time to devote ourselves to other things.

There are two basic principles in fasting. One is to add as much energy into our system as possible. Heat is energy, so we should add as much heat to our system as possible. The other is to stimulate our systems as much as we can. We can do that by using substances that slightly irritate, activate, awaken or mobilise it. Drinks during a fast can be water at room temperature or lukewarm, with or without lemon juice. You could also drink grapefruit juice in moderation. Another option is to drink stimulating (warming) herbal teas, such as ginger, cinnamon, fennel, nettle or ginseng. There are useful herbal products on the market that are advertised as "blood cleansing", "liver cleansing" or "intestinal cleansing". If the strong taste of stimulant herbs is a problem to you a spoonful of honey can be added once the infusion has cooled.

Try not to waste energy. This means that during your fast you should interact as little as possible with the outside world. Your intention must be on a different approach to life. You should not plan any strenuous physical or mental activity. You have to be aware of your own needs and feelings during your fast, allowing them to occur and attending to them. It is advisable to use a hot water bottle to provide warmth to sore areas, or simply to assist in the overall healing process. The neck, shoulders, lower back, and abdomen are areas where you might apply extra heat.

Movement will help your energy flow better. If you feel good during your fast, and only as long as you feel good, you can go for a walk, bike ride or swim (being careful not to lose heat!). All physical activities should be done calmly, never in a forced way. You have to adapt to how you feel in your system is at any given moment.

Breathing is a very efficient way to energise the system. Full yogic breathing is an ideal exercise for achieve this. During your fast you should spend a lot of time practicing this breathing technique. The very awareness of your breathing, slow and deep, in all circumstances of your life, will help you to lead a calmer life.

Ideally, you should extend your fasting period until you feel your system is ready to start digesting food again. If you don't have time to wait for that signal, I advise a minimum of three days of fasting. It is important to break your fast slowly and gently, so you can build up the energy you will need for digestion. You should start with foods that are as light as possible, as they require less energy for digestion. The best choices to start with are soups.

After that, for a period of two weeks, you should follow a very different eating routine from before the fast - no more than two small meals per day, always vegetable-based. Everything you ingest, including drinks, should be simple. Nothing should be eaten between meals.

How would you organise foods from lightest to heaviest to digest?

- Water and foods diluted in water, for example soups.
- Plants: plant-based foods, but not modern vegan "substitute" foods.
- Fish.
- Poultry, including eggs.
- Mammals: meat and dairy products.

You can "lighten" foods by cooking, which makes them easier to digest. Fruit is cold and not easy to digest, especially during the winter, but it is easier to digest when cooked. Generally speaking, your diet should consist of regional, seasonal foods.

A fast should be a time of contemplation. You should live in the moment and accept whatever you feel as part of who you are. You don't have to try to "make things better". You simply have to be. Your only reactions to your changing bodily sensations during the fast should be deciding whether to lie down and rest or whether to try moving gently. Your only concern should be to get yourself a hot water bottle as soon as you need it. The intention is not to change the circumstances, but to slightly alter the experience of the circumstances. This is how you change the focus.

The lasting effects of fasting are achieved by the change of focus. If you maintain a different outlook on life, as you experience during your fast, your mind and body will function differently. The fact that you become aware of aspects of your life that are putting stress on your system will provide you with the opportunity to make different choices when responding to the same circumstances. Reducing the influence of those situations and relationships that continually create tensions, and reducing the speed and pressure of life will result in your system functioning more efficiently.

Fasting helps cure diseases and, more importantly, helps to prevent them. Fasting is the true preventative medicine.

I have no doubt that fasting is the best preventative medicine, but you must admit that fasting at home is not easy, neither is staying in bed during an illness when it would be "so easy" to take painkillers or anti-inflammatories instead. Perhaps a good way to be able to exercise inner power would be to stay in a suitable place where it is easier to fast and rest, in the company of like-minded people. In the old days there were sanitoriums, in nature, where one could go and spend a few weeks or months to recover one's health, with good simple food, pure water, sun, nature. and good company. This was time to think and reflect, far away from daily life. Do you think that this would be a desirable health model?

 Indeed, not so long ago, every religion, every culture, had its "retreat centres", be they monasteries, temples, convalescent homes, sanitoriums or health spas. These places were not only accessible to all social classes but were places where people would stay for a considerable time to rest, recuperate and heal. They were mainly located near special natural places, such as springs, mountains or caves. Nature became the focus of attention, and people believed that it was the healing power of these special places that helped them get better. In fact, it is removal from daily life that often leads to illness or exhaustion, that gives our bodies the opportunity to recover. Moreover, being cared for and looked after by others instead of having to take care of everything oneself, adds a great deal of energy to an individual system. Also, in places of retreat, people are more willing to meditate or pray, to take care of their mind and body and to purify themselves, although these practices are available everywhere.

However, in less than a century, Western culture has achieved the following:

- That people concentrate only on working, earning money – so that there is no more happiness without money.

- That people who do not work, temporarily or permanently, need to be kept busy with nothing left in life but their survival. No possibility for growth, for learning, for being an individual.

- That people can only be cured by artificial means and that natural sources of healing are considered scams.

- That people should hand over power over their own health to medical authorities who are the only ones who have the power to decide what should be done.

- That people who are unable to continue with their former lifestyles should be kept busy with "health" appointments, medical tests and ongoing assessments by professionals.

The result of all this is that people's lives revolve around the amount of money they earn, what they can afford. What they can do is determined and restricted by how much money they are being charged to cover their needs. As the government provides a "free health service" and, by contrast, more traditional treatments, which they now call "alternative health treatments" are expensive (these have also become big business!), it is clear which of these two possibilities most people end up choosing.

Yes, you are right in saying that we need a new wave of retreat centres where people can stay, meet with other people and reconnect with themselves to heal their own ailments. All we have to do is to provide suitable places for people who are willing to open their lives and hearts to care for their fellow men.

Let's imagine now that we are in a quiet and peaceful retreat centre, although we could also be at home, and we are fasting. We have the time and desire to focus and work on ourselves. What do you propose as personal work? Where do we start?

➥ What you should try to identify is the problem itself, i.e. what type of energy is damaging your personal balance. Then you can make relevant decisions. Difficult? Not really. In general, people have the impression that there are thousands of possible influences to which they can be subjected, and therefore it seems a difficult task to identify what may be harming us. However, do remember that the entire universe is made up of only seven types of energy, which means that there can only be seven types of influences we must be aware of and evaluate. We have explained these in detail in chapter 5. I suggest rereading it calmly before tackling these questions as your personal work. When you find the type of energy that is harming you, you will know in which area of your life you need to take action. What you choose to do is up to you. If you can write the answers down, so much the better. Writing down the answers you have identified will be an extra help. Writing thoughts down requires a different set of neurological connections, which will help to "engrave" the knowledge in your memory bank and increase your understanding of the subject. Besides, you can go back to the answers again and again if you get lost along the way.

Go for it!

HOW TO BEGIN QUESTIONING YOUR OWN LIFE

1. Background/formation

How did your family guide you when you were growing up? What are the specific areas of conflict between your way of seeing things and your family's points of view? Are you comfortable with the way your family members relate or related to each other, with the hierarchy that manifests or did manifest itself in your family?

Appreciate the conflicts, as it is important to learn from them in order to find balance in your being. This is because what you need and what you have been receiving may be two different things.

2. Movement/change

In which aspects of your life do you feel too limited? Where do you encounter difficulties or complications in your development? In which parts of your life do you need a stable base and in which parts is it vital for you to have freedom?

Appreciate any resistance to your development process, as uncontrolled growth leads to a drastically reduced production of fruits, benefits in your life. Resistance will help you to question every step of your development. In this sense, we are still teenagers striving for a little more freedom, although, fortunately, we are still constrained by the guidance of parents or other authorities.

3. Personal power

Constraints stimulate the increased strength you will need to overcome them. However, what happens when your personal power is not enough to overcome your resistance? Is it time to distance yourself from opposing forces? Do you know your strengths and weaknesses? Do you know how to protect yourself in your weaker areas?

Be aware that there is always a choice between putting up a fight and walking away from a situation. Don't think that one is easier than the other. Making serious decisions in life is always difficult for someone who has to choose.

4. Balance

Learn to know yourself better. Are you giving more than you can afford or taking more than you need? With which skills are you over-endowed and which are you lacking?

Appreciate your skills and accept your weaknesses. Your weaknesses show you that you cannot be alone in life, that you need help. Know your weaknesses and learn to accept help and support, over and over again, even when it turns out that you have been taken advantage of, in which case you have the opportunity to learn from how it happened. You must practice, again and again, to open yourself to others in order to learn to receive.

5. Communication

From our environment we can learn that there are more ways to communicate. Communication is not limited to words since, in nature, words have less priority on the scale of how to get messages across to others. There is no such thing as "bad" communication. There is, however, a lot of "misunderstood" communication. The most important part of communication is learning how to listen. Have you found the right ways to express yourself in your environment?

Thank others for communications you don't understand. Do not blame them but stay close to them. This is an effective way for you to learn "a new language".

6. Intuition

Do you feel that you overreact to impulses that you encounter? Are you hypersensitive to certain stimuli?

If those impulses that bother you are within the natural range or are an ordinary part of everyday, then you clearly need to work on reducing the strength of your reaction to them. If those impulses are actually excessive, you need to move away from the origin to protect your system. Be grateful for strong messages that come to you, as they provide you with the opportunity to become stronger in relation to such impulses. If the impact becomes unbearable, you need to consider distancing yourself from the source and/or to close appropriate doors.

7. Conscious knowledge

When should you use logic and when should you use intuition, feeling or sensation?

The part of life constructed by human beings is based on logic. Practical problems are best approached from the angle of logic rather than from the heart, from what you feel. However, for the most part we are nature and therefore we are flows of energy that follow their own laws, independent of human logic.

How can you then be sure whether you are making a decision from the "heart" or from logic? When you are faced with a decision about the direction your life should take, write down in one column all the reasons you can think of why you should do a certain thing and in another column all the reasons why you should not. Once you have many more reasons in one list than in the other, choose the one with the fewest. The longer list of reasons will show you the logical approach. If you want to make a decision based on your heart or on intuition, you should not follow logic.

Which decision do you need to make?

Yes, I should do it because: no, I should not do it because:

SUGGESTED EXERCISES

Here are three more suggestions for exercises.

Exercise for concentrating the mind

Lie down in a comfortable position. Once you are comfortable, decide you are not going to move at all for a period of time, whatever sensations you may be feeling, or whatever happens. Ignore all sensations and just concentrate on following the order you have given your brain, which is not to move.

Exercise for learning to relax in your daily routine

Whatever your position, lying, sitting or standing, become aware of the areas of your body that are tense. Feel where there is a lot of pressure, perhaps in your joints, your muscles or even in your deep tissues. Once you have identified it, without changing your position, concentrate on letting the tension disappear, on relaxing the area. Feel where the muscles are contracted and release the tension.

Exercise for relaxing tension

When you are very focused on a physical activity in which you are tensing your muscles, become aware of your breathing. After holding your breath, in that moment of intense concentration, let the air out, and then make yourself breathe slowly for the duration of the physical effort or for as long as your deep concentration lasts.

As to what you ought to do when you are ill, I seem to have found, in the present discourses, all that is suitable: that is, that the surest remedy and the most favourable antidotes in any curable disease are *diet, quietness, time* and *tolerance.*

The Universal Panacea is composed of these four ingredients or, to put it more clearly, the All-Healer. And he who knows how to make use of it, will recover his health with little expense and will be cured with less danger.

Let everyone then think of the various things that may happen, of putting oneself in the hands of the physician; for he who will be deceived in the choice of the latter, will be deceived in the whole.

And so I repeat again:

Noli stultus ese, ne moriaris in tempore non tuo.

(Ecclesiastes. Ch. 7)

Do not be foolish, lest you die at a time that is not yours.

Yesterday and Today.
El mundo engañado por los falsos medicos
Extract from the book